P9-CSE-700

The Breast Cancer

Prevention Diet

ALSO BY ROBERT ARNOT, M.D.

The Best Medicine
Dr. Bob Arnot's Guide to Turning Back the Clock
Dr. Bob Arnot's Revolutionary Weight Control Program

With Charles Gaines

Sportselection
Sportstalent

Vanessa Wynn

THE BREAST CANCER PREVENTION DIET

*The Powerful Foods, Supplements, and Drugs
That Can Save Your Life*

ROBERT ARNOT, M.D.

LITTLE, BROWN AND COMPANY
Boston   New York   Toronto   London

Copyright © 1998 by Robert Arnot, M.D.

All rights reserved. No part of this book may be reproduced in any form or by any electronic or mechanical means, including information storage and retrieval systems, without permission in writing from the publisher, except by a reviewer who may quote brief passages in a review.

First Edition

Library of Congress Cataloging-in-Publication Data
Arnot, Robert Burns.
   The breast cancer prevention diet : the powerful foods, supplements, and drugs that can save your life / by Robert Arnot. — 1st ed.
      p.   cm.
   Includes index.
   ISBN 0-316-05114-4
   1. Breast — Cancer — Prevention.   2. Breast — Cancer — Diet therapy.
   I. Title.
   RC280.B8A76   1998
   616.99′44905 — dc21   98-20432

10   9   8   7   6   5   4   3   2   1

MV-NY

Book design by Barbara Werden Design

Published simultaneously in Canada by Little, Brown & Company (Canada) Limited

Printed in the United States of America

To the women in my life, especially my wife, Courtney,
my mother, Mary, and my three sisters,
Bonnie, Jeanne, and Nancy

Contents

Contents

PART THREE
BREAST CANCER PREVENTION PLANS

Acknowledgments

I would like to thank at the outset the dozens of leading organizations, hundreds of dedicated scientists, and thousands of brave women who have pioneered the concepts behind breast cancer prevention. In particular I'd like to thank the following individuals who gave generously of their time to the undertaking of this book:

Dean Ornish, M.D., America's greatest pioneer of self-help disease prevention, for his support and encouragement and for his original work with cancer prevention.

Ernst Wynder, M.D., president of the American Health Foundation, for the vision to see, research, and promote the role of nutrition and nutritional therapy in cancer.

Dr. Ken Setchell, Ph.D., whose name is synonymous with the development of soy as a powerful means of primary prevention.

Terry Shintani, M.D., who pioneered and developed the idea of multicultural cuisines as a means of treating illness.

John Glaspy, M.D., of UCLA for his brilliant work on

Acknowledgments

omega-3 fats and his infectious enthusiasm and dedication to his patients.

David Rose, M.D., of the American Health Foundation, for laying out so much of the groundwork for breast cancer prevention through diet.

Pat Murphy of the Iowa State University of Science and Technology for the most comprehensive consumer information on soy.

Leslie Bernstein, M.D., of the University of Southern California, for her creative work on estrogen and breast cancer.

Bill Helferich, of the University of Illinois, for his generous assistance.

Scott Grundy, M.D., of the Texas Health Sciences Center in Dallas, for first advocating changing fats as a health strategy.

Deborah McCurdy and Kathy Owens for being such brave and enthusiastic volunteers in UCLA's breast cancer prevention program.

Jack Fishman, M.D., and Leon Bradlow, M.D., of the Strang Cancer Prevention Center, New York, for their pioneering work in cruciferous vegetables and cancer.

David Jenkins, M.D., of the University of Toronto for discovering and warning us about the dangers of "glucose load."

Jon Michnovicz, M.D., of the Strang Cancer Prevention Center, New York, for his enthusiasm and for alerting us to the dangers of bad estrogens.

Rita Mitchell, R.D., and Barbara Sutherland, Ph.D., of the University of California at Berkeley, Department of Nutritional Sciences, for their enthusiasm and their tireless assistance in preparing the menus for this book and ensuring the menus are true to the principles of the breast cancer prevention diet.

Dr. Irwin Rosenberg, M.D., of the Jean Mayer Nutrition Center at Tufts University in Boston for his measured sense of decency and honesty and for his inspiration.

Dr. Pamela Goodwin for her breakthrough research on insulin and breast cancer.

Dr. Sam Epstein for so clearly laying out the dangers of chemical estrogens.

Mark and Virginia Messina for their work on soy and for their gracious assistance in helping us better to understand soy and how to use it in a rich and varied dietary program.

Lenore Kohlmeier, M.D., of the University of North Carolina for her wide-ranging work on human nutrients and breast cancer.

William T. Cave, M.D., of the University of Rochester for his leading role on insulin growth factor and fatty-acid metabolism and breast cancer.

Dr. Zora Djuric, Ph.D., a breast cancer specialist at Detroit's Barbara Ann Karmanos Cancer Institute, for her work on oxidative load.

Moishe Shike, M.D., Director of Clinical Nutrition, Memorial Sloan-Kettering Cancer Center, for his practical touch and well-founded skepticism.

Robert Pritikin of the Pritikin Longevity Center in Santa Monica, California, for pioneering the healthful low-fat diet.

Acknowledgments

Banoo Parpia of the China-Cornell-Oxford Project for her fascinating multicultural studies of breast cancer.

Walter Willett, M.D., of the Harvard School of Public Health for changing the paradigm of modern nutrition.

Dr. Lilian Thompson of the University of Toronto for laying out an entirely new dimension in breast cancer prevention.

John P. Pierce, M.D., for his farsighted breast cancer prevention diet.

Dr. Ercole Cavaliere of the Eppley Institute for Research in Cancer at the University of Nebraska Medical Center, for his new insight into the role of estrogen metabolites.

I'd also like to express my gratitude to the following institutions whose support, research, and funding are moving us all closer to the prevention of breast cancer.

Susan G. Komen Breast Cancer Foundation, one of the nation's largest private fund-raisers for breast cancer research, for all they have done to educate women about the risks of breast cancer.

The Cornell University Program on Breast Cancer and Environmental Risk Factors of New York, for its singular efforts in understanding the effect of environment on breast cancer and for its wonderful newsletter, *The Ribbon*.

The Harvard School of Public Health Department of Nutrition.

The University of California at Berkeley.

The Jean Mayer Nutrition Center at Tufts University in Boston for the most far-reaching efforts to establish the nutritional causes of breast cancer.

Memorial Sloan-Kettering Cancer Center for its innovative breast cancer prevention trials.

The H. Lee Moffit Cancer Center in Tampa, Florida, for its work on the breast cancer prevention diet.

The National Cancer Institute for its leadership in the prevention of cancer through foods.

The Strang Cancer Prevention Center, New York City.

The U.S. Department of Defense for its substantial funding of breast cancer research and for pulling together so many of the world's leading breast cancer specialists.

The University of California at San Francisco.

The China-Cornell-Oxford Project on Nutrition at Cornell University in Ithaca, New York, for the most fascinating and helpful look at cross-cultural nutrition.

The Barbara Ann Karmanos Cancer Institute for its work on oxidative load and dedication to women at high risk for breast cancer.

The U.S. Department of Agriculture for its excellent food-data tables.

The University of California at San Diego for its clinical research on a vegetable-based breast cancer prevention diet.

I'd also like to thank the following for their help in making this book possible:

Sarah Crichton, my publisher at Little, Brown, who had the vision to see how quickly breast cancer prevention would become possible.

Bill Phillips, my editor at Little, Brown, whose keen mind and analytical skills made this book eminently more readable and interesting!

Acknowledgments

Rima Canaan, my editorial associate, for her energetic help with the final editing and finishing touches.

Dan and Simon Green, my agents, for their hard work and determination.

Mary Wagner, my dedicated researcher, who, like a great detective, tracked down every last research paper on breast cancer prevention.

Part One

NUTRITION AND BREAST CANCER

INTRODUCTION

For decades, breast cancer has stood alone among major diseases, because its victims lacked even a single practical preventive measure with which to protect themselves. In most epidemics, we've had the power to defend ourselves: vaccines for the flu, lowered cholesterol for heart disease, smoking cessation for lung cancer, lowered blood pressure for stroke, and safe sex for AIDS. But despite the decades-long, terrifying increase in new breast cancer cases, women have stood virtually powerless to prevent the disease. That had left a quiet sense of desperation among survivors like 37-year-old Deborah McCurdy, mother of four. Deborah had advanced breast cancer that required four cycles of intensive chemotherapy, aggressive radiation, and a bone marrow transplant: "My little girl was only two. I had to live to see her grow up."

Deborah finally has a chance to do just that. The good news is this: In the spring of 1998 there emerged the first real hope for women like Deborah that breast cancer might be prevented. Years of investment in breast cancer research is finally beginning to pay off and yield major discoveries by leading scientists working in North America and Europe in nearly a dozen different scientific fields. Most of these discoveries were unveiled in bits and pieces and so are virtually unknown to the public at large, with little drawn together into a comprehensive plan. What appears is a great untold secret: Nutrition is emerging as the most important way to prevent breast cancer.

Deborah McCurdy is a firm believer: "What we eat is such a big part of our lives, there just has to be some effect from what we eat on how we get sick. It seems so logical."

Deborah is trying to prevent a recurrence through a unique breast cancer prevention diet at UCLA. As it does for every woman interviewed for this book, a breast cancer diet gives Deborah a remarkable sense of finally being in charge: "Having a sense of control made me feel more positive about my condition. I was able to make a difference and help myself."

Whether you're trying to prevent breast cancer or are a breast cancer survivor, you too can grasp that sense of control and hope that this disease can be prevented and its intensity diminished.

As a medical journalist, I confess that I was unaware that diet played any significant part in breast cancer until I was asked what seemed like a simple question: "How do I prevent breast cancer?" The question came from my wife, chairman of the associates committee at Memorial Sloan-Kettering Cancer Center. She rarely talked about it, but breast cancer had struck her mother at an alarmingly young age. Courtney and I had been through much of the catastrophe with her mother, from the first shock at the small mass on the mammogram, through the false hopes that the cancer would be contained, through the aggressive treatment, a mastectomy, to the new hope after reconstructive surgery, and now the endless, just-below-the-surface anxiety that this cancer could recur at any time.

Her mother is not alone in her anxiety. Courtney has stood powerless under the looming shadow of this dreaded disease wondering if — or when — it will strike her. Courtney is at a higher risk for early breast cancer due to her mother's young age when first diagnosed and several other risk factors. In her thirties, she already has annual mammograms. The clock is ticking, and she and I want the answer now. How do you prevent breast cancer?

I tell friends I have one of the most exciting jobs in the world. The greatest thrill is finding cutting-edge research that has immediate benefit in people's lives. Thanks to thousands of incredibly dedicated medical researchers who are willing to share their findings, I have access to critical, often lifesaving information months before it becomes public knowledge. Because nutrition as a means of preventing cancer has been such a neglected field, researchers have been unusually forthcoming — willing to share information that otherwise might take years to reach the public. In pursuing an answer for Courtney, I stumbled onto a quick succession of remarkable findings clearly connecting diet to breast cancer.

The first clue came while I interviewed Dr. John Glaspy of the prestigious UCLA Comprehensive Cancer Center. He had just published a study in the *Journal of the National Cancer Institute* about diet and breast cancer. John sounded like he had struck gold. For many women he had. What he discovered was breathtaking.

Like most breakthroughs, John's work was grounded in basic science. He knew that rats implanted with human breast cancers quickly developed fast-growing tumors when fed a diet heavy in omega-6 fats such as corn oil, safflower oil, and many brands of margarine. He also knew that cancers shrank quickly and dramatically in rats fed omega-3 fats, such as fish oils. Armed with this evidence, he asked a group of breast cancer survivors to ingest large quantities of fish oils.

We all think of preventive efforts as taking many decades to come to fruition. Kids are told "Eat your vegetables." Why? If we were truthful, we'd answer: "So you don't get sick in middle age" — not the kind of answer that gets much play with a nine-year-old. What Dr. Glaspy found amazed him — dramatic changes in three short months. The actual structure of these women's breasts had changed and had become far more resistant to breast cancer. After hearing his story, I asked John: How do you prevent breast cancer? I could feel his energy and enthusiasm practically lift the telephone receiver out of my hand, despite the distance of nearly three thousand miles. He said that the wrong diet was the major driving factor behind breast cancer in this country. John pointed out that we can learn from studying other cultures. For instance, breast cancer strikes one in forty Asian women compared to one in eight American women. Why? John believes the difference is a hugely beneficial diet. Foods aren't just a small risk factor for breast cancer, they can be nearly the whole game. John continued: The right foods may be the major driving force that curbs the current epidemic, accounting for as much as 75 percent of the risk of breast cancer. I thought about Dr. Glaspy's conversation for weeks afterward. Gee, if the cancer has already begun, isn't it too late to stop it? Sure, I was a big believer in foods as drugs — but drugs *that* powerful?

My next clue came from Dr. Dean Ornish. He was visiting my NBC office to talk about an amazing new project. Dean had become world-famous for proving the impossible — that heart disease could be not just stopped, it could be *reversed*. My jaw gradually dropped as he explained his newest quest — reversing cancer. He didn't mean reversing a cancer that was full grown but rather reversing the cancer when it was at its very youngest stages. Could it possibly work? He had preliminary proof which cannot be reported here until it has first appeared in a scientific journal.

Dr. Lilian Thompson from the University of Toronto has provided the most compelling early proof that cancer can be reversed. Her work is just now being prepared for publication. What she has found is that breast cancer size actually decreases with a daily course of flaxseed. Flaxseed is quickly becoming one of the most popular health foods in America and has been called one of the most remarkable healing foods of our time. Flaxseed has two critical parts, flax oil, one of the healthiest fats you can eat, and a special fiber that protects against breast cancer and heart disease. This breakthrough study shows that breast cancer size decreases in the short time period between the diagnosis of breast cancer and surgery. That phenomenon is uncommonly seen even with very powerful chemotherapy. But for food to cause a cancer to shrink, this is a real and remarkable first. That kind of shrinkage may reduce the surgery required from a mastectomy to a lumpectomy. Begun early enough, it might prevent cancer altogether.

That led me to an old friend of mine, Dr. Irwin Rosenberg. He runs the world-famous Jean Mayer Nutrition Center at Tufts University in Boston. I asked him: How can we possibly discover all we need to know about foods that prevent breast cancer now — not ten years from now. It was really a rhetorical question. I didn't honestly expect any answer but the usual — "we'll have to wait until the completion of randomized double-blind controlled trials." Those are the gold standard in medicine. There were a dozen such trials now under way to prove that diet prevented breast cancer, but they were years from completion.

However, I had guessed wrong. That was not Dr. Rosenberg's answer. He said: "Bob, most Americans don't want to wait. We have dozens of terribly promising preventive treatments for which the controlled trials have not been finished. But we have a new way of looking at the problem. It's called evidence-based nutritional analysis."

In his kind and professorial way he carefully explained that by piecing together all of the available data, we might find an answer. He was rapidly assembling a team to look at the available information for a variety of illnesses. I quickly turned to breast cancer, where there was already a wealth of nutritional evidence: from test tubes, animal studies, and human studies to studies on women in countries with low breast cancer rates — you name it. And the results of these studies weren't just a series of isolated facts but were all pieces of a giant jigsaw puzzle that could be put together. Very few pieces were still missing. By prodding researchers in the field, I might see those last few pieces fall into place. Evidence-based medicine, as reported in the *Journal of the American Medical Association,* involves "integrating current best evidence." Evidence-based nutritional analysis is why thousands of American women are already on a breast cancer prevention diet, women like Kathy Owens who have volunteered to be part of this brave experiment. Says Kathy, "I had the opportunity to work with scientists, people who actually know what works. It was a chance to help myself and to help other people. After you've had breast cancer, you want to help yourself, but you also want to help others, so they don't have to go through what you did. You get to help in some way by being in this study. It's a chance to give back, at the same time helping yourself become healthier."

Her physicians have integrated the very best from literally thousands of first-rate scientific papers on breast cancer. Taking a cue from Dr. Rosenberg, I understood that women didn't have to wait for all these long-range studies to be completed. Kathy could make a bet with the odds greatly in her favor that modifying her diet would go a long way to preventing a recurrence of breast cancer. "I was in a really negative situation, having breast cancer, but this is something positive that's come out of it. I've changed my diet, taken steps to help myself. It works. The study showed that and I know I feel better. I have some control again over my life."

The breast cancer prevention diet presented here will integrate all of the latest and most vital research for you into a diet that could save your life. I'm asking you to bet that this diet can play a large part in decreasing your risk of developing breast cancer or, if you already have breast cancer, preventing a recurrence. This is not a bet made on blind faith. It's a bet made on a sound analysis of all the current nutritional research. How good a bet is it? How safe a bet is it? Is it a bet you should make? Here's the case for making the bet today.

THE BREAST CANCER PREVENTION PILL WORKS

In April 1998, in a breathtaking discovery, the National Cancer Institute reported that high-risk women who took the drug tamoxifen decreased their risk of breast cancer by 45 percent. Tamoxifen diminishes the effect of estrogen, the chief fuel for breast cancer growth, by blocking the estrogen receptor — the key principle of the breast cancer prevention diet. For some very high-risk women, the breast cancer prevention pill will be an appropriate measure at the proper age, as we'll see in Part Three of this book. But for most women, the breast cancer prevention diet offers the benefits of medication but none of the risks, such as those of blood clots or uterine cancer. The breast cancer prevention pills, tamoxifen and raloxifene, are described at length in the chapter "Step 1: Block the Estrogen Receptor."

IT'S A BET BEING MADE WITH HARD CASH

Tens of millions of dollars are being spent on divining the nutritional secrets of breast cancer. Research dollars are invested incredibly conservatively. There must be milestones at every step of the way that show progress is being made — and it is in spades. Every piece of evidence points to a strong nutritional role — from studies of women in foreign countries with low breast cancer rates to studies of animals, test tubes, and humans. If the trail had turned cold at any step along the way, the cash would have turned off. It hasn't.

INTERMEDIATE END POINTS ARE KNOWN

Researchers look for "end points" in clinical trials. For breast cancer those end points would be fewer cases of cancer, fewer cancer deaths, less spread of the disease. Most studies are not that far along. There are, however, what are called intermediate end points. We can use these intermediate end points to evaluate the benefits of the diet; and the diet has already proved to be effective — it changes the breast's composition, and in some cases decreases the size of an already existent breast cancer.

YOU CAN'T AFFORD TO WAIT

The fully tested breast cancer prevention diet is a decade away. Why? Human nutritional trials take a very long time to do. For conclusive results, at least 1,000 women at very high risk would have to be studied for five years or longer. And the government won't fund most studies that don't concentrate on one single change, such as a low-fat diet. That means, at the end of those five years, there would be proof that only a single ingredient or nutritional concept worked, such as soy protein or fruits or vegetables. That's why constructing an entire program now makes so much sense. The breast cancer prevention diet provides an ideal framework with which to observe and incorporate changes in your diet as they are reported.

HEALTHIER BREASTS

Clear healthful fluid courses through the milk ducts of a healthy breast, capable of withstanding the insults of toxic foods and chemicals in our environment. However, in women who smoke or eat a high-fat diet that fluid turns dark and may contain toxins that increase the risk of cancer.

THIS IS AN EPIDEMIC, AND IT MAY ONLY GET WORSE

Since 1940 there has been a 1 percent increase per year in the rate of breast cancer. This epidemic is not just American, it is evident throughout the world and is increasing from Japan to Africa. In fact, breast cancer is the most common cause of cancer death for women worldwide. That means that your risk may continue to increase. The National Cancer Institute reports that there is no evidence of an epidemic. However, an epidemic is defined as an unacceptably high level by current world standards. In the case of breast cancer, rates are up to ten times higher in the United States than in Far Eastern countries.

IT WORKS FOR BILLIONS OF OTHER WOMEN

In the United States, out of 100,000 women, 30 to 40 are expected to die of breast cancer. In Thailand and Sri Lanka, that number is an astonishing 2 to 5! You could make the argument that the difference in numbers is due to genetic differences, but it isn't. When Asian women move to the United States, they and their daughters suffer an increased risk of breast cancer close to that of American women. When women move from countries with a high breast cancer risk to that of a lower one, their risk declines as well. It is diet and physical activity that protect billions of women in Japan, China, Korea, Thailand, and Africa.

YOU CANNOT ERR WITH A HEALTHY DIET

One could argue that a wait-and-see attitude would be prudent. That would be true if there were substantial risks in such a diet. However, the major error you would be making would be *toward* a much healthier all-around diet. The nutrients in the breast cancer prevention diet have been widely shown to prevent a host of other diseases, from heart attack and stroke to other major cancers, diabetes, and obesity. You can only improve your health.

IT'S A BET MADE BY THOUSANDS OF AMERICAN WOMEN WITH BREAST CANCER

John Glapsy has found the volunteers in his study to be the most dedicated patients he has ever known. Perhaps they've caught his infectious enthusiasm. Perhaps too, it's because his ideas really work. Kathy Owens says doctors "threw the book" at her in the summer of 1995. She underwent chemotherapy, lumpectomy, mastectomy, stem cell transplantation, and radiation therapy. "Tomorrow's my fiftieth birthday," she said when we spoke. "When I was diagnosed, I didn't think I'd be here to see it, so I'm celebrating, and I feel that I'm going to be around for many more because of the things that I'm doing, the changes that I've made."

IT BOOSTS THE EFFECTS OF BREAST CANCER PREVENTION DRUGS

Even the best estrogen receptor blockers don't entirely prevent breast cancer. The addition of a great diet adds tremendous synergy to decrease even further your risk of cancer.

FOOD IS A LOT KINDER TO YOUR BODY
THAN DRUGS

Drugs strongly interfere at one very specific point in the sequence that causes cancer, and can therefore develop prominent side effects. By changing your diet, you can interrupt many places in the sequence without the toxicity of drugs.

With the amazing inspiration of Kathy and Deborah and dozens of other heroic volunteers, I resolved to embark on a journey for my wife. We would spread all the research out on our dining room table like the pieces of a jigsaw puzzle. I would take as long as it took, turn over every last stone and come back to her with an answer. Since that resolution, I have combed the scientific literature from around the world, read thousands of papers, and visited the laboratories of the most prominent scientists at the finest scientific institutions, from Harvard and UCLA to the National Cancer Institute. Courtney and I have experimented with hundreds of different foods and food combinations at home. I have found dazzling new techniques for probing the nutritional secrets of cancer prevention. In the end we have uncovered the key elements of a breast cancer prevention diet. The diet is everything we imagined it could be and more — capable of quickly and effectively changing the actual structure of the breast, capable of changing the flow in the body of hormones that induce breast cancer from the very first day. It's a fun diet with lots of variation and many other benefits, from preventing heart disease and building stronger bones to losing unwanted body fat. But first and foremost it is a diet that will make you feel the best you have ever felt. This diet is carefully designed to lift your mood rather than dump it — as is so common when you're asked to give up the food you love. You'll also find this is a highly satiating diet that will make it far easier to shed unwanted fat. What you will find in the following chapters is a full account of the foods that cause breast cancer and the treasured foods that prevent breast cancer. You'll also find laid out a range of diets:

- a diet for women with high estrogen levels, i.e., those who have not reached menopause
- a diet for women with low estrogen levels, i.e., for those who are past menopause
- a breast cancer survivor's diet
- an intensive intervention program for women at high risk, using several powerful supplements
- dietary guidelines for your daughters; the earlier your children start, the better their chances of entirely avoiding this cancer

The breast cancer prevention diet is true primary prevention, but it does not displace secondary prevention — finding tumors at their earliest stages. That means that self-examination and mammography will still play a critical role in cutting your risk of death from breast cancer.

WHAT MAKES

BREAST CANCER

GROW

THE MYTH OF THE EUREKA FACTOR

Many of us in medicine have been brought up to believe in the "lone gunman" theory of breast cancer, which suggests that a single event or toxin or food "causes" cancer. You will read hundreds of news accounts over the years of foods linked to an increased risk of breast cancer. There have been lots of suspects, ranging from a high-fat diet and red meat to pesticides in foods, but they all have disappointed researchers. Why? What these researchers *really* want to find is a food that increases the risk by 500 percent. That would constitute a Eureka factor . . . a factor that almost certainly *causes* breast cancer. But unfortunately, none of these ever eked out a risk much more than 20 or 30 percent — very unimpressive numbers. That has caused many scientists and doctors to give up on finding or pursuing a breast cancer diet.

How then can food's role in cancer development be explained? The answer is that many factors have to be added together to develop and grow a breast tumor. These factors are not simply thrown together into a toxic soup. They fall neatly into place as part of a pathway that causes cancer cells to divide and grow. There is not one food that causes cancer but a well-defined series of foods that participate. Like a series of dominoes that need to fall, one onto another, a chain of events needs to occur before a cancer can grow. This chain reaction is set off by surprisingly few foods and can require only a few steps to blunt or block it. That's because these factors can create an astounding synergistic effect. Where one nutritional factor may have little influence, several together may exert a very damaging effect or a very powerful protective effect. "A favorable change in risk cannot be attributed to a single factor. A change in a woman's entire dietary pattern is probably responsible for reducing risk. That is, a diet high in fiber, fruits and vegetables and exercise, and low in fat and alcohol consumption," explains Steven Clinton, M.D., of Harvard's Dana Farber Cancer Center.

As an example, in rural South Africa, women have a breast cancer risk of four per 100,000, about 90 percent less than American women. They have a moderately low-fat diet, lots of fiber, and a modest number of calories. Each of those factors alone has little influence and has failed to produce any results in American women. But all three of these protective factors linked together yield remarkable, virtually unbeatable results.

This chapter lays out the chain of events that leads to breast cancer. As you will see there are only about half a dozen *steps*. That's good news, because as we've seen in rural South African women, every step is a potential target for prevention with the right foods — and the great news is that foods DO target each step.

Cancer development is divided into two stages. The first is cancer initiation, when a genetic mistake turns a cell cancerous. The second is promotion, which causes this cancerous cell to divide, grow, and spread. Since foods exert their most powerful effect on blocking cancer promotion, let's consider that first.

CANCER PROMOTION: THE ESTROGEN EFFECT

Breast cancer is called a "hormonally driven" tumor. That means the development and growth of the tumor is spurred by the body's hormones. In breast cancer, it is the hormone estrogen that primarily drives its development and growth. On balance, estrogen is an enormously healthful hormone.

We know estrogen primarily for its effect on the secondary sex characteristics in women, from growth of the uterus and thickening of the vaginal lining to breast development. Estrogen also has a variety of roles that promote great health. Estrogen protects the heart by making more good cholesterol and less bad cholesterol as well as keeping blood vessels pliable so they don't stiffen with age. Estrogen protects against bone loss by helping to absorb calcium from the bloodstream. In the urinary tract, estrogen helps to maintain the outer membranes of the urethra and bladder to prevent infections. Estrogen stimulates water retention and oil lubrication in the epidermis, so that skin remains soft and youthful. Scientists are just beginning to learn that estrogen interacts with nerve growth factors to protect brain cells from degenerating. Estrogen has been shown, in animal studies, to increase the number of connections between brain cells responsible for thought, movement, instinctive response, and learning. It also helps the brain to imprint new memories.

Although we talk about estrogen as if it were a single hormone, there are actually several different forms of estrogens. As you read this book, the key definitions to keep in mind are those for strong and weak estrogens, good and bad estrogens, and chemical estrogens. Estradiol is referred to as a "strong estrogen" in this book. This is the principal estrogen and is the most powerful natural estrogen produced by the body. There are also "weak estrogens" that counterbalance "strong estrogens." "Weak estrogens" are also called "plant estrogens," since these come from soybeans and flaxseed. The Strang Cancer Prevention Center in New York City has also popularized the idea of "good" and "bad" estrogens. As you'll read, estrogens become "good" or "bad" as the body prepares them for excretion from the body after their useful life is finished. One excretion pathway makes "good" estrogens, the other makes "bad" estrogens. This is explained at greater length in the chapter "Step 3: Make Good Estrogens." For now it's important to remember that there are both strong and weak estrogens and good and bad estrogens. The strong and weak are the active estrogens that circulate in the bloodstream. Good and bad estrogens are waste products. Chemical estrogens are just that, chemicals found in the environment, especially pesticides, that act like real estrogens in the body. Finally, there are "anti" estrogens. These are drugs, such as tamoxifen and raloxifene, that completely block the effects of estrogen in the breast.

All estrogens have one feature in common, they must lock on to a receptor to work. Receptors are "switches" that turn biological systems on, as an electrical switch would turn a light on. There are several critical differences. First is that the receptor is turned on only by a molecule that precisely fits the receptor, like a key into a lock. In this case, the key is estrogen. Recall the different-shaped blocks children play with, which have different-shaped matching holes to put them into: round, square, rectangular, for example. Think of an estrogen receptor as being a triangular hole. Only triangular-shaped estrogen of precisely the same size will fit. A square or round block would have no chance. That means that estrogen can fit into the receptor but other kinds of hormones cannot.

Estrogen works its widespread wonders because the brain, bone, skin, heart, uterus, and dozens of other body parts have these estrogen receptors. So with so many wonderful qualities, how could estrogen ever be considered harmful? There is one other body part, loaded with estrogen receptors that soak up estrogen from your bloodstream. It is the breast. When too many strong, bad, or chemical estrogens reach these receptors in the breast, the potential for cancerous growth rises.

ANATOMY OF THE BREAST

The mature female breast is made up of millions of tiny milk-producing sacs. Milk flows from these sacs into milk ducts that carry milk to the nipple. These milk-producing sacs and the milk ducts have an inner lining. Picture for a moment the ceramic tiles that might line the walls of a tunnel or an ancient aqueduct. Like these ceramic tiles, a special cell called an epithelial cell lines the inner surfaces of the milk sacs and milk ducts through which the milk passes. This, as we'll see, is the breast's Achilles' heel.

WHAT ESTROGEN DOES

Estrogen directly affects these epithelial cells that make up the milk sacs and ducts in the breast by attaching to their receptors. It is in these milk duct cells that cancer develops. Estrogen causes these cells to divide more often and more rapidly, creating thousands of new cells. It does this by turning on many genes responsible for growth and proliferation. Each time these cells divide there is the chance for a mistake to be made, leading to cancerous changes in the cell. Lots of estrogen causes these cells to divide, multiply, and grow even more quickly. It does this by speeding up the cell's "cycle clock." That is, each cell has a gene clock that dictates how quickly or slowly it grows and replicates itself. Lots of estrogen speeds up this clock. If these are cancerous cells what they need to divide and flourish is fuel, and that fuel is estrogen.

Let's follow the estrogen pathway from the time estrogen is produced, along its journey through the bloodstream to the estrogen receptors and its eventual effect on DNA. Remember that foods can powerfully block every one of these processes. We'll see how in the following chapter.

EXCESS ESTROGEN

The ovaries, adrenals, and fat cells are the key estrogen factories. If their production goes into high gear, large amounts of estrogens are secreted into your bloodstream and that increases your risk of breast cancer. Let's look at the evidence. Researchers at New York University measured estrogen levels in women long before they ever developed breast cancer. Years later the NYU Women's Health Study found that those postmenopausal women who developed breast cancer had a markedly higher amount of estrogen measured in their blood than those women who did not have cancer. A study of Chinese women showed that the higher their estrogen levels, the higher the risk of breast cancer. Also, American women with a family history of breast cancer have higher levels of estrogen. Now look at the protective effect on women who produce very little estrogen. Women who underwent total hysterectomies before age 40 had a striking 75 percent lower incidence of breast cancer. Since the ovaries were removed, their body produced very little estrogen. These are just a few examples. In all, there are nearly a hundred good studies that associate high estrogen levels with a high risk of breast cancer . . . and low levels with low risk. How much your risk of cancer rises also depends on the kind of estrogen that attaches to the estrogen receptors in the breast. Let's now look more closely at the different kinds of estrogens that can increase the risk of breast cancer.

Strong Estrogens

Consider that estrogen, represented as a triangular block, has to fit into a triangular receptor. Think of that block as a battery. The strongest estrogen, estradiol, may carry the power of a big car battery — greatly increasing the risk of cancer. Why? When estradiol attaches to the estrogen receptor it creates a powerful signal inside the breast cell for cell growth. Other estrogens might carry the power of a small penlight battery. Weak estrogens might have the power of a very small camera battery. The more powerful the estrogen, the greater its cancer-promoting potential. Very weak estrogens may actually protect against cancer by blocking access to the receptor, so powerful estrogens cannot insert themselves. In essence, all of the triangular holes get filled up by the weaker estrogen, leaving no more space for the powerful estrogens. That means very little power is delivered to the cell and the signal that reaches the cell's DNA is weak, creating very little potential for cell growth.

Chemical Estrogens

Natural and plant estrogens aren't the only ones that can attach to breast receptors. So can certain synthetic chemicals. Pesticides in our food and water, called chemical estrogens, can mimic the biologic actions of estrogen. That's because they have the same "triangular" shape as natural estrogens made by the body. They are so similar in their molecular composition to natural estrogens that the estrogen receptor can't tell the difference between them. These chemical estrogens lock right into the estrogen receptors and stimulate cells in the milk ducts to divide and grow, just as real estrogens do. Although there are only minute quantities of these pesticides in our food and water, the breast can concentrate them to highly toxic levels. How? As we've seen, the breast is constructed from milk duct cells that are surrounded and supported by fat cells. These fat cells can concentrate chemicals to toxic levels. For instance the breast fat cell absorbs a form of the pesticide DDT from the bloodstream and stores it at concentrations 700 hundred times greater than is found in the blood.

Bad Estrogens

At the end of the day, estrogen is discarded by the body. To make estrogen easier to dispose of, the body changes estrogen into different forms. But which disposal form your body makes may determine whether or not you get breast cancer, according to researchers at the Strang Cancer Prevention Center in New York. The breakdown products are a "good" estrogen or a "bad" estrogen, much like the "good" and "bad" cholesterol in your blood. The good appears to protect against breast cancer, whereas the bad may play a very powerful role in triggering the development of cancer. Foods can increase the amount of "good" estrogen you make. Among Japanese women who had breast cancer, those with high counts of "good" estrogen had no spread to the lymph nodes. Among those who had low counts of "good" estrogen, there was spread to lymph nodes. Later in this book you will find an entire chapter on good and bad estrogens.

Recycled Estrogens

Estrogen circulates through the bloodstream for less than a day, then is disposed of by the body, which transports it from the bloodstream through the liver and into the bowel for excretion. Once estrogen is put into the bowel for disposal, you'd think that was the end. Unfortunately, estrogen can be absorbed from the bowel into the bloodstream, which can contribute to higher estrogen levels in the blood. This happens when there is too little fiber to bind estrogen and carry it from the bowel.

Free Estrogen

Most estrogen is transported from the ovaries and other production sites in the bloodstream on what is a called a carrier molecule. You might think of the estrogen as a triangular log tightly strapped onto a barge for transport down a river, rather than floating freely in the river by itself. Only estrogen that is "free" can attach to an estrogen receptor in the breast. The higher the amount of "free" estrogen in your blood the higher the risk of breast cancer. Estrogen cannot make its way into the breast to attach to a receptor so long as it is attached to its carrier. The technical name for the carrier is sex hormone binding globulin, or SHBG. As we'll see, binding more of the free estrogen by building more carriers is a significant way to lower your risk.

Anti-estrogens

These are drugs such as tamoxifen and raloxifene. They dramatically cut the estrogen effect, blocking access of all estrogens to the estrogen receptor so that there is no signal for growth inside the breast cell.

PROLONGED EXPOSURE TO ESTROGENS

High levels of estrogen are only one way to increase your risk. The other is to increase the total amount of time you are exposed to estrogens over the course of a lifetime. The more years you menstruate, the greater your risk of cancer. Both an early menarche and a late menopause create years of increased estrogen exposure. Girls with the earliest menarche, before age 14, have a 30 percent increased risk of cancer. Women who have a later menopause, say age 55, have a 50 percent higher risk of breast cancer than those whose menopause occurs before age 45. The most fascinating evidence comes from Catholic nuns studied in Europe over 300 years ago. These nuns had a markedly higher level of breast cancer than married women with children. They obviously weren't being studied at the time for estrogen levels, or in any systematic, scientific way. But in hindsight we recognize the cause of their cancer was the uninterrupted estrogen flow.

BOOSTING THE EFFECT OF ESTROGEN

After estrogen has completed its journey from the ovaries through the bloodstream to the receptor, the game is far from over. The only way estrogen works is by attaching to a receptor. Once estrogen attaches to the receptor, the signal can be magnified enormously to create a strikingly higher risk of breast cancer. This is called a "booster" effect. That means, whatever power estrogen carries to the receptor, that power can be magnified so that the final effect on cell growth is tremendous. As we'll see, the kinds of fats you eat determine the amount of booster effect.

CANCER INITIATION: PULLING THE TRIGGER

So far we've seen the role of estrogen as a fuel that causes cells to divide and grow. But something must still "pull the trigger" to initiate changes in the cell that turn it cancerous. When scientists say they are looking for the "cause" of breast cancer they are really looking for whatever substance or toxin damages the cell's DNA. DNA is thought of as an extraordinary blueprint that carries all of the instructions for the complete building, care, and maintenance of every part of the human body. But DNA goes beyond mere blueprints; it is also chief architect and general contractor, manufacturing the elements that build every element of every cell in the body.

The entire complement of DNA contains the equivalent of 500,000 typewritten pages. Imagine having those half million pages on a computer disk and having the disk constantly zapped by chaotic electrical surges, 24 hours a day, 7 days a week, year in and year out for 80 years — without ever suffering a single misspelling or loss of data — while being used by tens of thousands of computer operators. Error-free operation is just not possible and that's the trouble with DNA. It's under a blistering daylong attack. These blueprints get zapped up to 1,000 times every day by the toxins that are in our environment and in the foods that we eat. To protect itself, DNA has an enormous repair crew to repair the damage. This repair crew has to spot that one error out of a billion and fix it. Should, however, the repair crew get taken out of action by potent carcinogens — or should the damage be so devastating that it can't be repaired — the damaged DNA reprograms a normal cell and turns it into a cancer cell.

Doctors have classically been led to believe that there is just a single "zap" that pulls the trigger and creates an error that leads to cancer. With breast cancer, nothing could be further from the truth. The new emerging concept is that there are *lots* of mutations and genetic defects. For the most benign of cancers, there are at least half a dozen errors. For the most severe and aggressive, there are up to 50 errors. Each one may come from a different cancer-causing substance. When scientists look at DNA, they see a distinct pattern of damage that is characteristic of environmental damage. The gene most frequently damaged is called P53. But the distinct patterns of damage vary widely from one population of women to another. So it's likely that women in Austria suffer a very different kind of damage than women in Los Angeles or Australia. Thus it is very difficult to come up with one approach to preventing cancer initiation. But there is one new emerging concept — an overall measure of the daily siege that DNA undergoes. It goes by the name "oxidative load."

"Oxidative load" sounds fairly innocuous, but here's what it means. Elements in the body called free radicals are responsible for the cellular damage that occurs with aging, in heart disease, cancer, and most degenerative diseases . . . regardless of what the original toxin may have been. These free radicals cut and hack away at DNA at a furious pace. The more free radicals clustered around doing their damage to your DNA, the higher the "oxidative load." Inside your body they are created from fat metabolism. External sources range from solar and ionizing radiation to cigarette smoke, air pollutants, heavy metals, ozone, organic solvents, pesticides, and food additives. More to the point, researchers can actually see a higher oxidative stress in the breasts of women with breast cancer than in those who are cancer-free.

So, in summary, while we can't single out specific foods or toxins that initiate breast cancer, we can measure oxidative load. The lower that load, the lower your risk of cancer, and certain foods dramatically reduce oxidative load. The following chapter looks first at how to cut the estrogen effect and then at how to lower oxidative load.

HOW FOODS

CAN PREVENT

BREAST CANCER

CHEMOPREVENTION

There have been four standard ways of treating cancer: radiation, chemotherapy, surgery, and biological therapy. Now emerging is a new and far more important technique, chemoprevention. Chemoprevention allows you to prevent a cancer from growing in the first place or to treat a preclinical cancer. Many of you are familiar with this idea from Pap smears that have come back abnormal but not cancerous. They may show "dysplasia" but not cancer. Early treatment prevents cancer. We know that a breast cancer could take as long as 33 years to develop. For much of that time it is unseen and undetectable by standard methods. As an example, in their forties, 40 percent of women have small cancers in their breast that escape detection, according to autopsy reports of women who died from other causes. Only when the tumor reaches one *billion* cells in size can a mammogram detect it; that's the smallest that a radiologist can see but it is simply enormous in terms of cancer growth. What this book is designed to do is change the biology of your breast so that you create a very unfavorable climate for a cancer to grow. Here's how.

Cancer is often treated with a variety of chemical agents to target the cancer's life cycle in as many ways as possible. Because of our great daily familiarity with foods, we tend to discount their ability to work as medicines. But look at the proven ways in which foods can act to target cancer development. They can:

- disrupt hormonal pathways that cause cancer
- repair the genetic material DNA
- inactivate harmful chemicals
- inactivate enzymes that drive chemical reactions
- scavenge mutant cells
- lower oxidant levels with antioxidants
- inhibit tumor growth

— basically the entire tool chest needed to stop a cancer before it starts. And fighting cancer requires a big tool chest.

This chapter will show you how you can block the estrogen effect in a step-by-step fashion with the right kinds of foods. Remember that the key principle of cancer chemotherapy is to use several different agents to interrupt the cancer cell's growth with several critical choke holds. The same concept applies *before* a cell becomes cancerous, using multiple agents to block the amount of estrogen that flows through the bloodstream and attaches to estrogen receptors in the breast.

You will find that many of these steps can be targeted with more than one nutritional strategy. Some of the same strategies such as high-fiber or low-fat diets affect more than one step because they have more than one anticancer action. You'll find each of these measures covered at length in a chapter of its own. There's a lot of science in this chapter. Don't be overwhelmed by it. In the end, it all comes down to blunting the estrogen effect and blocking the trigger that causes cancer. As you'll see in the last part of the book, the diet itself is pretty simple. I include the science because knowledge leads to tremendous empowerment and because it will allow you to change and adapt your diet as new discoveries are made. The more you know about what you are doing to your body, the more likely you are to succeed.

SLOW DOWN ESTROGEN PRODUCTION

How useful is the idea of decreasing the effect of estrogens? R. L. Prentice, in *Cancer Causes and Control,* estimates that a 17 percent reduction in the key estrogen, estradiol, might produce a four- to fivefold reduction in breast cancer. In other words, small changes in estrogen levels can effect large changes in the risk of cancer. Let's look at the most effective steps.

Low-Fat Diet

A low-fat diet is eaten in those countries, such as China, Japan, and Singapore, with the lowest incidence of breast cancer. Countries with higher-fat diets — these include England,

Scotland and Wales, and Finland — have more breast cancer. For instance, Finnish women on higher-fat diets had higher estradiol levels than Asian women — and far higher breast cancer rates. In fact, if there is one common denominator found in Asian women with low risk of breast cancer, it is a low level of estradiol. Remember that estradiol is the most important and powerful of the natural estrogens. A high-fat diet increases estradiol production by 30 percent. In dozens of animal experiments, a high-fat diet spurs the growth of cancers. But the connection between low fat and low estrogen levels isn't just an observation, it is something that works in real life. The *British Journal of Cancer* showed that a 15 percent low-fat diet, followed rigorously for two years, lowered estradiol levels by 20 percent.

High-Fiber Diet

Hand in hand with a low-fat diet is a high-fiber diet. Americans pay great lip service to fiber but eat vanishingly little of it by world standards. However, when the American Health Foundation made a real effort to increase fiber intake substantially, even they were surprised by the results: The more wheat bran patients ate, the lower their blood levels of estrogen were. After just two months of a 20-grams-per-day wheat bran supplement, estradiol decreased significantly. But the addition of high fiber to low fat is especially potent medicine. African-American women have far higher levels of estrogen than Caucasian women. Their high-fat, low-fiber diet is held accountable. Doctors at Tufts University fed African-American women a 40-

grams-per-day high-fiber diet combined with a 20 percent low-fat diet. Estradiol fell 8.5 percent and estrogen sulfate, the most prevalent estrogen, fell by 22 percent. This same high-fiber, low-fat diet works wonders for millions of women trying to control excess body fat.

Lower Body Fat

Excess body fat works as an enormous estrogen factory. The more fat cells and the bigger they are, the more estrogen they produce. As many women gain weight, those who gain it "up top," that is, in their breasts and upper abdomen, add the greatest risk. Obesity is associated with poorer survival in women who contract cancer. The less body fat you have, the less estrogen you will produce. When studying Japanese women, scientists hypothesized that a big part of the reduced risk of cancer they see in a low-fat diet simply comes from having less fat and therefore less estrogen. Keeping body fat low is especially important as an adult. Weight gain from early adulthood may account for as much as a third of new cases of postmenopausal breast cancer.

Lower Insulin Levels

Only recently has a connection been made between insulin and breast cancer. Insulin is a strong promoter of the estrogen effect. Insulin is like half-strength estrogen, stimulating cells to divide just like estrogen. That may sound unimpressive, but estrogen and insulin work synergistically, stimulating DNA to copy its messages for cell growth and division. It is yet another example of how one and one adds up to far more than two. A high insulin syndrome often depends on where you store fat. If you have an "apple" shape, where excess body fat is carried above the hips, you are at risk for a high insulin level. That's contrasted to the "pear" shape, where excess fat is carried below the hips in the thighs and buttocks. A diet rich in starches and sugars increases insulin levels. This is referred to as a high-glucose-load diet. Because your system cannot handle the tremendous "load" of sugar that this diet pours into your system, your body will pour out equally large amounts of the hormone insulin to defend itself. Women who gain body fat around the upper abdomen usually eat a high-glucose-load diet and suffer from an excess production of insulin. Since high insulin level is such a potent promoter of the estrogen effect, it's important to cut those insulin levels both to protect yourself against cancer and to control your weight. The chapter "Step 4: Lower Insulin" tells you how.

Limit Alcohol

Whether you produce a moderate or high amount of estrogen, alcohol is one last factor that can drive any amount of estrogen to an even higher level. Alcohol is fast emerging as a major risk. The risk of breast cancer is increased 11 percent per drink per day. Four drinks a day and your risk increases 44 percent.

Aromatase Inhibitors

These drugs can cut the production of estrogen from fat stores in the breast to nearly zero. They are soon to be used in clinical trials to prevent breast cancer.

DECREASE OTHER ESTROGENS

Here's how to counter the ill effects of bad, recycled, chemical, and free estrogens.

Bad Estrogen

Even if you produce moderate to high amounts of estrogen, there is an emerging strategy to blunt its potency. You can actually channel your estrogen into good estrogen rather than bad estrogen by eating a diet high in cruciferous vegetables. Those include cauliflower, broccoli, and cabbage. Both exercise and low body fat also increase the production of good estrogen. Alcohol, polyunsaturated fats, and too much body fat all increase the production of bad estrogen.

Recycled Estrogen

When estrogen is transported from the bloodstream through the liver and into the bowel for disposal, it is assisted by large amounts of fiber in the bowel. That fiber binds to estrogen in the intestine so that the body cannot reabsorb it, ensuring that it is excreted with other waste products. However, when there is too little fiber in the diet, the estrogen remains free in the bowel and may be reabsorbed by the body into the bloodstream, raising the amount of estrogen in the bloodstream. A study at Tufts University showed that the more a woman's bowel movement weighed, the lower was her blood estrogen level. The assumption is that the increased weight of the bowel movement was due to the fiber.

Free Estrogen

The most effective way to decrease the amount of free estrogen in the blood is to build more of the carriers that bind estrogen in the blood and keep it from estrogen receptors. Let's look at the key strategies. The prime regulator of estrogen carriers is the hormone insulin, according to Banoo Parpia of the China-Cornell-Oxford Project. The lower you can drop your insulin, the more estrogen carriers your body manufactures. A low-fat diet also reduces the amount of free estrogen in healthy postmenopausal women. Soy also manufactures more carriers. A high-fiber diet helps to bind more free estrogen in your blood and keeps it at lower, safer levels. Many of these measures also decrease estrogen production, so you are cutting your cancer risk in at least two separate ways.

Chemical Estrogen

The most aggressive prevention includes avoiding animal and fish products with high fat contents that can pick up and concentrate large quantities of chemical estrogens and pesticides. The worst offenders and how to avoid them are found in the chapter "Step 8: Avoid Chemical Estrogens." Eating organic foods that have always been pesticide-free will help you to avoid contaminating breast fat. Washing all fruits and vegetables thoroughly will help remove pesticides. Since most women already have high stores of chemical estrogens in their breast fats there are two other strategies that have proved to be beneficial. First is breast-feeding, which flushes pesticides out of their storage site in breast fat. That does mean that your infant ingests milk with chemical estrogens, but pediatricians do not believe this is harmful. The most practical strategy of all is to consume large amounts of estrogen blockers such as soy, which block the effect of these chemicals at the estrogen receptors on breast cells.

SHORTEN EXPOSURE TO ESTROGEN

Decreasing the total number of days that you are exposed to estrogen substantially decreases your risk. There are two potential ways of doing that. The first and most practical is to change the length of your menstrual cycle. Asian women have longer menstrual cycles than American women, 33 days instead of 28. Why is that important? If you have longer menstrual cycles, you will have fewer total cycles over the course of a lifetime. Fewer cycles means less exposure to estrogen. Can you lengthen your menstrual cycle? Dr. Ken Setchell, a pioneer in the use of soy protein, gave a group of American women 60 grams of textured soy protein daily. He was able to prolong the cycles of these women to 33 days, mimicking the longer cycle length of Asian women. Vigorous exercise also decreases the total number of lifetime menstrual cycles by lengthening the menstrual cycle.

Some doctors, such as New York University's Steve Goldstein, prescribe birth control pills for longer than the usual 21 days in order to achieve a longer cycle. Newer birth control pills that could increase cycle length to prevent breast cancer are in the planning stages. With the decrease in numbers of childbirths and in years of breast-feeding, women today may have over 200 more menstrual cycles than their forebears. All this extra estrogen exposure may account for a substantial part of the increased risk of breast cancer that American women face.

The second method of shortening estrogen exposure is to delay menarche, since the more years you ovulate, the more menstrual cycles you will have. Young women with menarche before age 14 have a 30 percent increased risk of breast cancer when compared to girls whose menarche is at age 15 or later. Girls eating high-calorie, high-fat diets who undertake little physical activity have earlier menarche than active girls on lower fat, more modest calorie intakes. Young women in rural China on a low-calorie, low-fat diet with lots of physical exercise don't reach menarche until age 17. The later menarche occurs, the lower estrogen levels will be over a lifetime.

BLOCK THE ESTROGEN RECEPTOR

We've looked at how powerful estrogens that your body makes and chemical estrogens can act as "keys" that easily fit into the "lock" or estrogen receptor on breast cells. The most logical question to ask is this: "Gee, even if you produce too much estrogen, can't you just block that estrogen when it gets to the breast cell's receptor?" The answer is a resounding yes, you can block that tidal wave of estrogen *before* it gets to the receptor. This may be the most powerful and logical strategy of all.

It's a strategy that oncologists caught on to early. In fact the drug tamoxifen, given to early-stage breast cancer patients to prevent a recurrence, works exactly that way. Tamoxifen blocks the estrogen receptor. Evidence shows it works, providing 85 percent disease-free survival after five years in early-stage breast cancer patients. But tamoxifen is a powerful drug with significant side effects — not something you'd want to take before you got cancer. Fortunately there are foods that perform exactly the same function. They are plant-derived substances that mimic the action of estrogens and also fit into the estrogen receptor. However, they do not have the strength of estrogens made by the body and are up to 1,000 times weaker. This means when they fit into the estrogen receptor they bring little power to the receptor and so have little effect on the cell's DNA or on breast cell growth. When a large amount of these "weak" estrogens block the receptor, stronger estrogens and chemical estrogens cannot gain access. In this way, a large enough quantity of weak estrogens can greatly dilute the effect of all the natural and chemical estrogens. If weak estrogens occupied most of the estrogen receptors in the breast, the estrogen effect would be cut enormously. The two most important sources of weak estrogens are soy and flax, which are covered in the next chapter.

How protective are they? Premenopausal Chinese women had a 50 percent decrease in breast cancer rates on a high-soy diet. Keep in mind that these women already have 80 percent less cancer than American women — so that's a much more dramatic effect than you might expect. But the most stunning study to date is that of Lilian Thompson, who has been able to show that the tumors of women who've been diagnosed with breast cancer and who take flax for the usually short period between diagnosis and surgery, no more than several weeks, actually decrease in size!

BLUNT THE ESTROGEN SIGNAL

The other strategy involving the receptor is to weaken the cell's response to estrogen. Once estrogen locks on to the receptor, a signal is transmitted to the cell's DNA. The strength of that signal determines estrogen's final effect. A very strong signal can mean dramatic cell growth. A very weak signal can mean little growth at all. What determines that signal strength? The kind of fats you eat. Omega-6, found in safflower oil, peanut oil, soybean oil, and corn oil, causes a very powerful signal. In fact, omega-6 fats have been shown to increase the growth of breast cancers in multiple test-tube and animal experiments. In humans omega-6 fats account for a stunning 69 percent increased risk of breast cancer. That's the bad news. The great good news is that you can replace these omega-6 fats in your body. Here's how. First, avoid all omega-6 fats. You'll find a complete list in the chapter "Step 2: Change Fats." The next step is to eat a diet high in omega-3 fatty acids, which are found in fish oils. Studies of the breast fat in American women in California show almost no omega-3 fats at all! The omega-3 fatty acids in fish oil have a very positive effect on breast cells by cutting the signal strength dramatically. The other beneficial fat is an omega-9 fat, the kind found in olive oil. Olive oil is a neutral fatty acid. It doesn't have the toxic effects of omega-6, nor does it have the beneficial effects of omega-3. Yet the fact that it replaces omega-6 fatty acids makes for a net positive effect because the signal strength is reduced. Breast cancer rates are 50 percent lower in Mediterranean countries, where far more olive oil is used on salads and for cooking, than in the United States.

PROTECT THE BREAST DUCTS

The milk ducts of women who have never given birth are considered immature, which puts them at a higher risk of developing cancer than women who have lactated. When breast tissue matures, it becomes hardened to the effects of cancer-causing substances. That's precisely what soy protein does in younger women — matures the breast ducts to make them more cancer resistant.

Can you blunt the estrogen effect too much? This phenomenon is unknown in human adult women. Chinese and Japanese women, who follow virtually every single step above, do not have known fertility problems as a result. One radical theory is that estrogen levels should be *very* low at all times except when you want to get pregnant. The amount of estrogen that still maintains youthful skin tone and body shape and healthy heart and bones is a good deal less than most premenopausal American women produce. Here, however, is the concern. Low estrogen levels cause a greater than 50 percent miscarriage rate in pregnant baboons, primates whose hormones during pregnancy act much like those of humans. The fetuses died before miscarriage. Given those studies, you should consult your obstetrician about the wisdom of reducing your efforts to cut the estrogen effect during pregnancy.

BLOCK THE TRIGGER

Large amounts of estrogen act as the fuel that can ignite a breast cancer. With the stage set, all that remains is to pull the trigger and turn a cell cancerous. How do you block the trigger? Eat a combination of foods that drop your oxidative load by supplying a large amount of *anti*oxidants. Lots of antioxidants cut oxidative damage substantially. The only effective way of ingesting those antioxidants is through a diet high in fruits and vegetables. Dozens of studies show that women eating more fruits and vegetables get less breast cancer. One of the most important, out of the Harvard School of Public Health, showed that women eating the most vegetables had 48 percent less breast cancer than those women who ate the least. Those eating the most fruits had 32 percent less instances of the disease.

As powerful as any of these individual steps may be, they will probably not prevent breast cancer by themselves. However, combining them can produce a powerful synergistic effect. The following chapters describe in great detail each of the strategies outlined here. Each section has a complete analysis of the foods described, the key scientific arguments behind their benefit, and a consumer section on dosing, safety, and actual products you can buy. Some of the steps are still highly experimental, others solidly proven and widely accepted. You may find, as we have, that you'll simply incorporate what you find in these chapters into your diet. If you'd rather have it all incorporated into a simple meal plan, you'll find those meal plans at the end of this book.

Part Two

12 STEPS TO PREVENT
BREAST CANCER

STEP 1: BLOCK THE
ESTROGEN RECEPTOR

Make no mistake about it, estrogen receptor blockers work. They block the estrogen receptor from the effects of estrogen and they do decrease the risk of breast cancer. Tamoxifen, an estrogen blocker, cuts the risk of breast cancer by nearly half in high-risk women. Raloxifene, another blocking drug, may cut that risk by 90 percent. We'll look at both of those in depth at the end of this chapter. Since we are only in the infancy of understanding who should take the breast cancer prevention pill and what the ultimate side effects of taking such a pill for decades might be, most women are looking for safer natural alternatives. We'll look at two, soy and flaxseed.

SOY

A thousands-of-years-old natural experiment is under way with an estrogen blocker called soy. Soy has the potential to be the most important superfood in the world today, with effects that range from keeping you alert and thin to protecting you from heart disease and cancer. Premenopausal Chinese women have about a 50 percent decrease in breast cancer risk when they consume high amounts of soy. Contrast that to Chinese women who consume soy foods less than once a week and have twice the risk of breast cancer. Premenopausal women in Singapore with the lowest risk of breast cancer eat 55 grams of soy per day and have less than half the risk of breast cancer of women who consume the lowest doses of soy. This is critical because these women already have a far lower rate of breast cancer than American women. A case-control study from Australia showed a significant reduction in pre- and postmenopausal breast cancer for those women eating high amounts of soy and other foods containing weak estrogens. That's also been observed in America in vegetarian women with high soy intakes, who also have lower risks of breast cancer.

Breast Benefits of Soy

Soy's role in cancer prevention is potentially the strongest described in this book simply because it strikes the estrogen pathway in so many places. The only kind of soy products that work to block the estrogen receptor are ones containing an ingredient called genistein. Soy products with no genistein had no effect on blocking the estrogen receptor. Genistein is the estrogen-like molecule found exclusively in soy that displaces much stronger estrogens and chemical estrogens from the estrogen receptor.

Soy also has a wide range of highly esoteric cancer-fighting effects that are independent of genistein. Soy helps to build more of the carrier that binds estrogen in the blood. Eating large amounts of soy decreases the density of breast tissue. Women I have interviewed who have been on a high-soy diet remark on a softer feel and texture to their breasts. Less dense tissue makes mammograms far easier to read, so an early diagnosis is possible.

SOY CONSUMER'S GUIDE

Dose

Once any food is used as a drug, doctors necessarily become much more concerned with dosage, and that is true of soy. Very large quantities, well over a hundred grams a day, loads your system with estrogens. Even though they are weak ones, they are nonetheless estrogens and enormous quantities may flood estrogen receptors and increase the estrogen effect. This would be especially true for postmenopausal women or children who do not naturally produce large amounts of estrogen. Too little soy may also show a proliferative effect, meaning small quantities may cause breast cell growth. This effect has only been shown in test tubes and animals — not humans. Nonetheless, if you are going to take soy, taking the proper dose is critical to obtaining the desired effect. This is described as a "window" with both an upper and a lower safe limit. In Asia, the average dose of soy is 35 grams a day. This is a pretty safe floor, or lower dose. Sixty grams is the maximum amount used in most clinical trials involving breast cancer patients.

The table on page 52 includes a short list of soy foods and the grams of soy protein they contain per standard serving.

PROTEIN CONTENT OF VARIOUS SOY FOODS

Soy Food	Grams of Soy Protein	Serving Size
Miso	11.8	1/2 cup
Natto	17.7	1/2 cup
Okara	3.2	1/2 cup
Soy flour, defatted	47.0	1/2 cup
Soy meal, defatted, raw	45.0	1/2 cup
Soy protein concentrate	58.1	1 ounce
Soybeans, cooked and boiled	16.6	1/2 cup
Soybeans, dry-roasted	39.6	1/2 cup
Soy milk	2.8	1/2 cup
Tempeh	19.0	1/2 cup
Tofu, raw, firm	15.6	1/2 cup
Tofu, raw, regular	8.1	1/2 cup

As you can see, consuming that 60 grams of soy is easier said than done, since you may end up needing to eat up to three pounds of foods — which brings us to soy shakes.

Soy Shakes

The easiest way to eat the large amounts of soy necessary to protect you from breast cancer is a protein powder–based soy shake. Add a banana, water, ice, and some soy protein powder into a blender, then drink it like a milk shake. As a powder the soy protein is more quickly broken down and absorbed. UCLA uses concentrated powders in its cancer prevention trials. They know each subject is getting exactly enough. Soy protein powder is available as Vegi Fuel from Twinlab or directly from the manufacturer, Protein Technologies. Nagi Kumar's study at the H. Lee Moffit Cancer Center in Tampa uses the Protein Technologies product. Dr. John Glapsy's study uses Take Care, an unflavored powder that can be consumed in a strawberry smoothie, in lemonade, or in a honey drink, chocolate shake, marinara sauce, chocolate chip cookie, soup, or muffin. This is the easiest way to be certain you're getting exactly as much soy as you choose. Three servings of Take Care daily contains roughly 60 grams of soy protein. It works great first thing in the morning as a waker-upper. Be sure to buy high-quality products such as those made by Protein Technologies and Twinlab. Other manufacturers may use alcohol extraction techniques that take out most of the genistein. You can determine the genistein content of the product you're using by closely examining the label or by asking your pharmacist.

Purists will want to eat traditional Asian soy foods as part of an Asian diet, since they are better digested and absorbed than many second-generation or "engineered" soy foods. You will really have to eat a great deal of soy, however, to ingest the equivalent of 60 grams of soy protein. If you choose to go this route, the food plans in Part Three of this book list a variety of simple soy-based meals. The most practical soy food is the soy nut.

Roasted Soy Nuts

Soy nuts provide an almost complete meal. A soy snack will fill you up and give you the alerting hit of a good protein. Soy is like the potato. Just as most of the potato's food value is in the skin, most of soy's mineral value is in the hull. The advantage of whole roasted soy nuts is that they retain the hull.

The newest trend, however, is soy foods engineered for taste and convenience.

Second-Generation Soy Foods

Food technologists at universities and food companies are scrambling to come up with better-tasting and more convenient soy foods. They've also decreased the pure bulk of soy foods. That's key, since consuming 45 grams a day of soy protein would require eating three pounds of tofu! Taste chemists and mouth-feel specialists start with crushed soybeans and aim toward a product that tastes terrific and is more convenient to eat than boiled soybeans.

The New, Improved Soy Burger

These have a true burgerlike mouth feel and taste but without the heavy, pit-of-your-stomach aftereffect. It's a great quick-hit meal in one, with lots of vegetables and soy. The White House orders Boca Burgers, which have nearly zero fat. Boca Burgers, manufactured by the Boca Burger Co., in Fort Lauderdale, Florida, are tasty soy burgers that come in three different flavors. They can be found at health food stores and discerning supermarkets. The genistein content of this product has not been made public.

Soy Milk

This has got to be the easiest way to consume soy protein and takes only a couple of days to get used to. You'll find soy milk refreshing, relaxing, and invigorating. Since soy milk is at the low end of genistein concentrations, you'll need to drink lots of it. Look for low-fat varieties, since normal soy milk has as much as four grams of fat per serving.

Engineered Soy Foods

Soybeans may be ground and then processed into a fine flour. Look for soy-based muffins, breads, bakery items, shakes, soups, even pretzels that are engineered to taste great. Be sure to look at the label. Beware of products that combine soy flour with lots of white flour or hydrogenated oils.

Textured Soy Protein

This is the product many veggie burgers are constructed from. It begins as soy flour that is compressed to give it a meatier, more granular texture.

These second-generation products have created a far greater appeal to Western taste buds, but are not as rich in genistein, the key active ingredient that blocks the estrogen receptor. For example, tofu yogurt and tempeh burger contain only 6 to 20 percent of the genistein contained in whole soybeans. The table following shows the amount of genistein in traditional soy foods as compared to that of second-generation soy foods. Only the tempeh burger contains a comparable amount of genistein. The table was prepared by Pat Murphy of the Iowa State University of Science and Technology.

GENISTEIN CONTENT OF SOY FOODS

Soy Foods	Genistein (micrograms per gram of soy)
TRADITIONAL	
Roasted soybeans	869
Tofu	162
Tempeh	320
Bean paste	245
Fermented bean curd	224
Honzukuri (rice and soybeans)	177
SECOND-GENERATION	
Soy hot dog	82
Soy bacon	69
Tempeh burger	196
Tofu yogurt	94
Soy Parmesan	8
Imitation mozzarella cheese	36
Fat noodle	37

Practically speaking, this means that you'll have to eat more of the second-generation products to get the right amount of genistein.

Be sure that whichever soy product you choose, it has enough genistein, the actual estrogen receptor blocker: 40 to 60 milligrams is the amount of genistein to aim for per day. The table in the Appendix lists the genistein levels for the most popular products.

X-Rated Soy Products

These products won't help you fight cancer.

Soy oils: The one form of soy that doesn't shine is as a vegetable oil. Soy vegetable oil contains 61 percent omega-6 fatty acids. Its hydrogenated form is even worse.

Soy sauce: I love the stuff but it has only a minuscule amount of soy protein. It's often loaded with sodium. If you rely on soy sauce for anything more than good taste, you'll be out of luck.

Genistein supplements: The breast-protective ingredients of soy can only be activated by bacteria in the intestine. Soy works its magic by its conversion in the gastrointestinal tract, which is why actually eating real soy food is so key. That means real foods work better than supplements. Be sure *not* to take genistein as a supplement by itself until more research is completed. Taken as a supplement — and there are about a dozen such products on the market — genistein can *increase* breast cell growth, in part because it is so easy to overdose on it. The other big concerns from overdosing are stunted growth and a loss of fertility. In the next year, the safety of genistein supplements should be resolved. Until then, you're better off sticking with soy foods and high-quality soy powders that fully extract all the key ingredients from soy.

Soy Boosters

Curcumin: The most powerful soy booster is curcumin. Dr. Barry Goldin showed that adding curcumin to genistein has a dazzling effect. Take estradiol, the most powerful estrogen. On a scale of 1 to 100, its potency ranks a 100. Add genistein and that potency drops to 31.6; add curcumin and it drops to 1.5! Curcumin significantly decreases the estrogen effect of several pesticides. Curcumin is also a potent anti-inflammatory agent, an anticarcinogen, and an antioxidant. It is the active ingredient in turmeric root. Turmeric, in liquid extract or powder form, gives Indian curries fragrance and flavor and has long been championed in India for its health benefits. Turmeric is widely available on the Internet and in health food stores and is an excellent spice for most vegetarian dishes. Indian turmeric is the best and comes in several popular varieties:

- "Alleppey Finger" and "Erode" turmeric (from Tamil Nadu)
- "Rajapore" and "Sangli" turmeric (from Maharashtra)
- "Nizamabad Bulb" (from Andhra Pradesh)

Vegetarian Diet

The digestive process is vital to activating the key ingredients in soy. That makes a complex-carbohydrate diet important, since it increases fermentation in the intestine, which activates the active ingredient in soy. Asians consume a higher percentage of complex carbohydrates than Americans, as well as less animal protein. This higher carbohydrate intake increases weak-estrogen absorption.

Side Effects

Just as the popularity of soy is reaching an all-time high, several researchers have warned that genistein is still a weak estrogen and that any estrogen could cause cell growth. One experiment looked at the growth of breast cells in a test tube. With no other estrogens, genistein could cause these cells to grow. As yet unpublished studies looking at fluid expressed from the nipples of women who took soy also show signs of breast cell growth. This does not mean that there is any risk of cancer with soy. To the contrary, thousands of years of use by billions of women shows exactly the opposite, a striking decrease in cancer. This research, however, makes many researchers reluctant to recommend soy until more is known. My own feeling is that soy is a good estrogen blocker for women who produce large amounts of estrogen. For postmenopausal women who produce low amounts of estrogen, the question is whether the introduction of even a weak estrogen will stimulate cell growth. For these women, there is less need for soy and so less need to recommend it. This is clearly an issue you'll want to follow closely in the news and discuss with your doctor.

Build Up to It

Soybeans can cause serious intestinal gas and discomfort, as can any food with high concentrations of soluble fiber. For that reason you will want to start with 10 grams a day of whole soy foods that still contain fiber and build slowly over a month. Since you may be eating these foods for years, don't start with an unpleasant experience. There are some people who have a food intolerance to soy and are unable to digest it at all. For them, the best alternative is flax. While soy has captured the spotlight as the primary dietary means of blocking estrogens, flax is quickly catching up.

FLAX

Flaxseed is one of only a handful of foods considered by the National Cancer Institute to be a designer food, that is, a food that has so many cancer-fighting qualities it's as if it were tailor-made as a medicine, not just a food. Curiously, flax is the only food noted in this book that blocks the estrogen pathway and the estrogen booster effect. That's because it contains that rare combination of a weak estrogen and an omega-3 fatty acid. It's so potent that researchers at the University of Toronto are treating women with breast cancer with flaxseed. The researcher Dr. Lilian Thompson is giving flaxseed to women at the time of diagnosis. As noted earlier, she has shown a decrease in tumor size in women taking flaxseed between the time of diagnosis and the time of surgery. You may feel somewhat shortchanged by the amount of material on flax. Whereas soy has been studied for decades as an estrogen receptor blocker and over a thousand scientific articles and scores of books have been written on it, flax is only now emerging as a factor in breast cancer protection.

Breast Protective Benefits

Flaxseed is the richest known plant source of omega-3 fatty acids and the richest source of weak estrogens, making it a true superfood. Flax can also limit the estrogen in fat cells, limit the booster effect, lengthen the menstrual period, and increase the number of estrogen carriers. That's nearly every step in the estrogen pathway. Pretty amazing stuff!

Dose: Lilian Thompson gives her patients 25 grams per day of brown flaxseed, ground and incorporated in a whole-grain muffin. Since the estrogen blocker is created by the bowel after digesting the flaxseed, only flaxseed, not oil, provides the proper estrogen-blocking effect. It is important that the seeds be ground — grinding breaks the seed's hard outer coat so that the human enzymes have better access to the beneficial elements inside the seed.

Following Dr. Thompson's example, you can grind flaxseed and incorporate it in your baked goods — breads, pancakes, muffins, or cookies. Use your coffee-bean grinder to grind the seeds.

You can also buy a variety of ready-made breads containing flaxseed. The table below lists flaxseed-containing breads available nationwide in health food stores or in stores such as Whole Foods Markets. If stores in your area do not carry a particular bread, call the bakery at the number listed to place an order.

As you can tell from the table of flaxseed breads, few commercially available breads contain enough flaxseed to give you the recommended 25 grams a day in just a few slices. An easy way to make sure you receive your daily 25 grams is to grind the

COMMERCIALLY AVAILABLE BREADS
WITH FLAXSEED

Whole Foods Markets

Bread	Grams of Flaxseed Per Slice
Flaxseed Bread Sourdough European Bakery 512-442-7879	5.06
Honey and Flaxseed Bread Bread and Circus Bakery 617-389-1324	3.5
Three-Korn Bread Sourdough European Bakery 512-442-7879	1.2
Honey-Grain Boule Bread and Circus Bakery 617-389-1324	0.88

flaxseed and incorporate it into other foods: Put it in your orange juice, sprinkle it on your salad, mix it in applesauce, cottage cheese, or yogurt — be creative!

You can usually buy bulk whole seeds: In her experiment, Dr. Thompson uses a brown flaxseed produced by Linott; other producers include A. C. Linora, Andro, Flanders, McGregor, Noralta, Norlin, Norman, Somme, and Viny. Arrowhead Mills widely distributes packaged flaxseed. You can also order the flaxseed from Heintzmann Farms in South Dakota (toll-free phone number: 888-333-5813 or 800-333-5813).

TAMOXIFEN

National Cancer Institute officials were described by my friend Larry Altman at the *New York Times* as "jubilant" when they proved tamoxifen could lower the risk of breast cancer for women at high risk. That's because their historic study provided the first major evidence that breast cancer could be prevented.

Women who took the tamoxifen had 45 percent fewer cases of breast cancer than a group of women who took a dummy pill. Remarkably, the drug worked in all age groups. That's the good news. The bad news is that tamoxifen can also kill you if you're over 50. While the number of new cases of breast cancer fell nearly by half, the numbers of new cases of cancer of the uterus nearly doubled. Women over 50 can also develop blood clots in their legs, which can work their way into the lungs, causing a life-threatening emergency. That's unfortunate because women over 50 are those who would benefit most. The greatest criticism of the study is that the federal researchers didn't wait long enough to determine if the drug actually saved lives — the ultimate end. Some fear that the drug might just delay breast cancer, rather than entirely prevent it.

Tamoxifen did have the added benefit of maintaining stronger bones but did not prevent heart attacks, as hormone replacement therapy would. Women in the study took 10 milligrams twice a day. Tamoxifen is not officially approved by the FDA for cancer prevention. The agency will review the data to determine who is best suited to take the drug. Even so, the number of women in America who qualified for the government's study was small: only 27 in 1,000 at age 40 and 93 out of 1,000 at age 50. Currently the FDA does not recommend tamoxifen to women unless they are part of a clinical trial. With all these problems, researchers say they hope for newer drugs. Fortunately, one of them is already here and it's called raloxifene.

RALOXIFENE

Presently, 10,000 women worldwide are enrolled in a raloxifene study designed to evaluate its role in preventing cardiovascular disease and breast cancer. At an open FDA meeting in November 1997, researchers presented interim data showing a stunning 77 percent decreased risk of breast cancer for women who have been on the drug only 18 months. Doctors inside the clinical trials report to us that the 30-month data are even better, approaching 90 percent. Dr. Brian Walsh of Harvard says that the final results will bring us to the cusp of an explosion in breast cancer prevention. What about side effects and risks?

Raloxifene does not increase the risk of cancer of the uterus even after 39 months of use. The reason is that raloxifene is a "selective" estrogen that blocks the effect of estrogen in the uterus as well as the breast yet has a positive effect on the heart and bones. The major risk of raloxifene is that of blood clots, but this risk is equivalent to what women who take hormone replacement therapy would expect.

You might well ask, if raloxifene is so good, why has tamoxifen generated all the excitement? When the National Cancer Institute began its trial, tamoxifen was the only estrogen receptor blocker available. Most researchers say that if the trials were begun today, a newer estrogen receptor blocker, in all likelihood raloxifene, would have been chosen. Gynecologists like NYU's Dr. Steven Goldstein are amazed at all the attention tamoxifen is getting, given that newer drugs are so superior. Who should take raloxifene? Postmenopausal women who are at high risk of breast cancer and for osteoporosis and who do not want to risk taking hormone replacement therapy should consider raloxifene and could start taking it today. They'll enjoy the FDA-approved benefit, prevention of osteoporosis, and an added secondary benefit, decreased risk of breast cancer. A University of California at San Francisco study has shown that it is safe in younger women, but the FDA cautions that raloxifene is not approved for use in younger women.

This is a terribly exciting time and we can expect to learn

lots more about the use of these drugs. Until it's determined which drug is best for you, the safest bet is to stick with food-based estrogen blockers that have stood the test of time, unless you are at very high risk for breast cancer. In that case, you should consider enrolling in a clinical study at a major cancer center.

One last question is, gee, if estrogen blocker drugs work so well, why bother with the diet? First, estrogen blocker drugs are too toxic for many women. Second, even for those women who do take them, they don't eliminate breast cancer risk. They intercept only a single point in the estrogen pathway. The recommendations in the rest of this book will allow you to intercept multiple critical points in the estrogen pathway to reduce your risk even further and to make the effect of estrogen blocker drugs far more powerful.

Recommendation

Include 35 to 60 grams of soy protein or 25 grams of flaxseed in your daily diet once you and your doctor agree on the appropriateness of the estrogen receptor blocker strategy for you. For women at very high risk, an estrogen blocker pill may be appropriate. You'll find more on these drugs in Part Three: "Breast Cancer Prevention Plans." Even for those women who take a breast cancer prevention pill, the features of this diet, found in the following chapters, add powerful synergistic effects.

STEP 2: CHANGE FATS

Fat has been the foremost suspect among all food elements in the genesis of breast cancer. But after a classic study of 350,000 women reported in the *New England Journal of Medicine* showed that the amount of fat in the diet just didn't make any difference, most serious researchers abandoned the hypothesis. As this theory died, remarkable new evidence has demonstrated that the kinds of fat you eat are far more important than how much fat is in your diet. Also, since most Americans are not willing to give up fat, there is a great deal of allure to simply changing fats. By doing so, you may strikingly alter the balance in your risk of breast cancer and heart disease.

WHY THE WRONG FATS ARE SO DANGEROUS

Milk ducts are surrounded and supported by fat cells. Look at these fat cells as supply depots. Whichever fat is stored in them is supplied directly to the milk duct cells. The fats they store are the fats you eat. If the fat cells contain healthy omega-3 breast fats, the estrogen signal in the cell is weakened. An omega-6 fat greatly increases the signal strength. Women have the added disadvantage of storing more omega-6 fats than men.

FATS TO AVOID

Omega-6 Fats

We know these fats by their more traditional name, polyunsaturated fats. They are found in most vegetable oils and margarines. One of the biggest changes in the diet during the years that breast cancer risk has risen has been the rise of omega-6 fat consumption. North Americans have shown the largest increase in consumption of vegetable oils in the world over the past 30 years. Doctors are just beginning to understand the dangers of omega-6 fats. They have proven dangerous in the test tube and in experimental animals. Few researchers realized exactly how powerful the booster effect was until the appearance of the January 12, 1998, issue of the American Medical Association's *Archives of Internal Medicine.* It reported in a study of 61,471 women that "polyunsaturated fat increased the risk of breast cancer by 69 percent." A previous Iowa study of 34,388 women showed a 50 percent increased risk with polyunsaturated fats.

A study of Greek women suggested an increased risk just from consuming margarines high in omega-6 fats.

The Western diet now contains up to 20 times as many omega-6 as omega-3 fats, or a 20:1 ratio. That ratio should be much closer to 4:1. For millions of years prehistoric women lived on a diet that was 1:1, closer to what we are genetically adapted to. You may say to yourself, gee, he's got to be kidding. I thought we were all encouraged to eat *lots* of vegetable oil and margarine as a way of preventing heart disease. That is true. We made a very bad trade a generation ago. In an effort to stem the tide of heart disease, public health authorities encouraged Americans to give up saturated fat for polyunsaturated fat. Unfortunately, polyunsaturated fats are the building blocks of the breast cell's booster system. Dean Ornish estimates that American women are eating 500 times the amount of omega-6 that is considered healthy. Harvard-trained Dr. Terry Shintani points out that hundreds of millions of women are in a large-scale experiment right now, taking huge quantities of omega-6 fats with all the attendant health risks. The American Health Foundation theorizes that omega-6 fats contribute to the metastasis and spread of cancer, whereas omega-3 causes a suppressive effect. That is solidly backed up by test-tube and animal studies. Now major nutrition department heads around the world believe that while omega-6 fats did contribute to the decrease in heart disease as a substitute for saturated fats, they also contributed substantially to the rise in breast cancer. "We chose the wrong fat," I have heard over and over again while writing this book. Many voice this opinion privately because they are waiting for more evidence, and they're right . . . not all the information is in yet. However, I firmly believe that you risk nothing by changing fats. You might ask if it's a trade-off, dropping omega-6 fatty acids to prevent breast cancer at the risk of developing heart disease. The answer is no. Omega-3 and omega-9 fatty acids are far more heart healthy than omega-6. You gain in preventing both diseases by eating omega-3 and omega-9 fatty acids. Whereas omega-6 simply decreases the bad cholesterol, omega-3 and -9 both decrease bad cholesterol and increase the good cholesterol.

OMEGA-6 FATS TO AVOID

Safflower oil

Corn oil

Soybean oil

Peanut oil

Cottonseed oil

Grapeseed oil

Borage oil

Primrose oil

Sesame oil

Foods made with omega-6 fatty acids:

> Mayonnaise
>
> Commercial salad dressings

Margarine

Transfatty Acids

The worst of all omega-6 foods are those that have been chemically altered into transfatty acids by a process called hydrogenation. This process makes potato chips crisper, shelf life longer, and the fat firmer. Researchers looking at the actual amount of transfatty acids stored in body fat found that those women who stored the most transfatty acids had a 40 percent increase in their risk of breast cancer. To avoid transfatty acids, don't buy foods with the words "hydrogenated" or "partially hydrogenated" on the label. These can reduce the production of the healthy prostaglandins. Good prostaglandins decrease the booster effect in breast duct cells. You will hear food companies loudly complain that these fats are as little as 2 percent of the diet. They are right. But here's the rub. Fat cells, including those in the breast, are thought to concentrate transfatty acids, so although your intake may be small, the amount in your breast may be high. The most obvious source of transfatty acids is stick margarine, which can contain up to 17 percent transfat. But most transfats are hidden from you, in commercial baked goods, French fries, fried foods, crackers, and cookies. Transfats' biggest risk is that of heart disease. By replacing the 2 percent of transfats in the diet, heart disease risk dropped 53 percent, as reported in the Harvard Nurses Health Study.

Saturated Fats

The major danger of these fats lies in their ability to increase insulin levels. The outer layer of your muscle is what allows sugar to pass into the muscle cell. However, if you have a diet high in saturated fats, that outer layer will pass sugar with a great deal more difficulty. That makes your muscle much more resistant to the effects of insulin, which will cause your blood fat levels to rise. The body then has to make more insulin, which increases the risk of breast cancer. Twelve case-controlled studies link a high saturated fat intake with breast cancer. Saturated fats are found in whole-fat dairy products, cheeses, and red meats. A high intake of saturated fats can also triple your risk of heart disease. If you do not have excess body fat, then these saturated fats may be eaten in moderate quantities: Game meat, chicken, eggs, chocolate, low-fat cheese, and butter blends with olive oil are the safest best. Fatty red meats are a different story.

Fatty Red Meats

A study of 14,291 New York City women found that those women who ate the very most red meat had a 25 percent increased risk of breast cancer. A case-controlled study conducted in Uruguay found an increased risk of red meat that ran from 230 percent to 770 percent. Curiously, the risk may come from animal protein itself. An Italian study showed a risk just from a high intake of animal protein even when the risk of saturated fats was subtracted. What's the safest bet? Studies do show a sharp *decrease* in risk with vegetable proteins. If you love meat and can't do without it, however, consider how it is cooked. All meats are likely to be of lower risk if they are marinated and not grilled over an open fire. Grilling can introduce a potent carcinogen called heterocyclic amines. Heterocyclic amines are thought to contribute to cancer development because they damage DNA and have been shown to induce tumors in animal studies. More heterocyclic amines are created when meat (as well as poultry and fish) is cooked at high heat (barbecuing, broiling, pan-frying) until well-done. Microwaving, boiling, stewing, or poaching produce less. Rare to medium contains fewer heterocyclic amines, well-done contains more — it's even in the gravy made from the pan drippings. The safe way to barbecue is to precook — microwave for 2 to 5 minutes, which releases juices that contain precursors of heterocyclic amines. Be sure to discard the juice. Another alternative is to precook in steam or in a low oven and finish cooking on the grill. Marinating is a great way to go. Although its not known why, researchers have observed that heterocyclic amines levels fell by 90 percent in barbecued chicken that was first marinated.

Refined Carbohydrates

You may not think of carbohydrates as fats, but that's the way they end up in your bloodstream. If you eat a very low-fat diet, high in refined carbos and sugars, your body will make a saturated fat called palmytic acid, one of the very worst. That's reflected in your blood as an increase in triglycerides, which carry fat in the bloodstream.

FATS TO EAT

The American Health Foundation reports that both omega-3 and omega-9 fatty acids reduce breast cancer risk. Omega-3 fats aggressively cut the effect of omega-6 fatty acids and help to quiet the estrogen booster effect in the cell. The most prominent foods containing omega-3 fatty acids are fatty, deep, cold water fish. (See the "Omega-3 Fats" chapter.) Omega-9 fats, best known as monounsaturated fats such as olive and canola oil, are covered in the "Omega-9 Fats" chapter.

THE RIGHT LOW-FAT DIET

What about just eating less fat? A low-fat diet has been the earliest and longest-lived candidate for breast cancer reduction.

As we've seen, those countries with the very lowest fat intake, such as China, have the very lowest breast cancer rates. Countries with the very highest fat intakes, New Zealand, the Netherlands, England, and the United States, have the very highest breast cancer rates. And when women in other countries actually increase the amount of fat they eat, up goes their risk of breast cancer. Higher fat consumption in childhood and adolescence can lead to faster growth and earlier menarche, both known risk factors for breast cancer. With the adoption of a higher-fat diet, even women in the Far East are suffering from a striking increase in breast cancer. In Singapore there has been a staggering 3.6 percent increase per year in breast cancer rates as women there change to a high-fat, low-fiber Western diet. The danger of high fat has been a very convincing argument. In the United States, however, the argument fell flat on its face. Fifteen years ago everyone thought a high-fat diet explained the high rate of breast cancer in America. Today they don't. When studies of dietary fat were done *within* the United States, no such low-fat connection was made. Researchers hoped to find a 24 percent decrease in breast cancer with a 25 percent fat diet. Instead, they found none. Why? Lowered fat content is just one ingredient. Women in Asia take advantage of all the other steps outlined in this book. Their diet has a low glucose load, is high in fiber, high in soy, and low in calories. Fat was just one small element. Look what happens when you add just one more ingredient, fiber, to a low-fat diet. Barry Goldin and Margo Woods of Tufts University report in the journal *Cancer* that a low-fat, high-fiber diet did decrease blood estrogen by 9 to 15 percent. Remember how the South African villagers whose diets were low-calorie, low-fat, and high-fiber had a strikingly low rate of breast cancer? A low-fat diet that is high in calories and omega-6 fats, low in fiber, devoid of soy, and has a high glucose load (the average American low-fat diet!) is likely to raise your risk of breast cancer.

The other major reason that the low-fat diet has not panned out in American studies is that no studies were really low-fat! Consider that Asian women are eating a 10 to 15 percent fat diet. The average American diet ranges from 34 to 43 percent fat! The biggest and best study of fat and the risk of breast cancer, the famous Harvard nurses study, had very few women who even dropped to a diet of as low as 20 percent fat. Also, most American studies have been too short to show more of an effect. Japanese and Chinese women eat low-fat foods in childhood, adolescence, and early adulthood. No American studies have tracked women since adolescence, when much of the benefit of a low-fat diet is evident. Breast cancer prevention pioneer Dr. Ernst Wynder, president of the American Health Foundation, is currently enrolling 1,400 women in a trial of a 15 percent low-fat diet to settle the issue once and for all.

There is only one real way to undertake a low-fat diet and that is to undertake a high-quality vegetarian diet. On a high-quality vegetarian diet, I would aim for 10 to 15 percent fat. Twenty percent is the upper limit recommended by most cancer centers. There is no real argument *for* eating a high-fat diet just because a low-fat one hasn't proven out in clinical trials. A diet high in saturated fats poses a high threat of death from heart disease. The choice is yours, the low-fat vegetarian diet of Asian women or the healthy-fat diet of Mediterranean women. Both strategies are described in the chapter "Healthy Cuisines."

FEWER CALORIES

One last reason a high-fat diet may be dangerous to good breast health is that it just has too many calories. Dr. Moishe Shike of Memorial Sloan-Kettering is the biggest fan of holding excess calories responsible for excess breast cancer. In fact a low-calorie diet protects against breast cancer. This is backed up by a large number of animal experiments that show that calorie restriction substantially decreases the number of breast cancers.

But there was also a highly unusual, unplanned human experiment, when food rationing was in effect in Norway during World War II. Girls born between 1930 and 1932 consumed far fewer calories than the previous and later generations. Those exposed to a virtual famine at about the age of menarche had a 13 percent decrease in death from breast cancer. This risk decline in breast cancer death continued even after menopause. A recent local study by the South African Institute for Medical Research revealed that the daily energy intake of five-year-old rural black girls was about 1,000 calories, compared with nearly double that amount in Caucasian girls. These black girls have a tiny fraction of the amount of breast cancer risk that the Caucasian girls have.

Don't you need a lot of calories if you have cancer?

Sure, for late-stage disease, many patients even require supplemental feeding. But at Sloan-Kettering, women without advanced disease seem to do better with a lower calorie intake. "If I had to recommend one measure to prevent breast cancer, it would be a low-calorie diet," says Sloan-Kettering's Dr. Shike. He recommends a diet of no more than 1,500 calories for most women. He even recommends a low-calorie diet to early-stage breast cancer patients as a way of preventing a recurrence.

The greatest folly is not to eat too little but to eat foods that are high in starch or fat and low in fiber and nutrients. Even with fewer calories, that diet is more likely to keep fat on and the risk of breast cancer high. You'll want to sit down with a nutritionist and plan how many calories to eat, taking into account your activity level.

Recommendation

There is a simple bottom line. You *do* want to give up saturated fats, transfats, and omega-6 fats. The best alternatives are either fish oils or olive oils. If you go the low-fat route, as I've said, choose a high-quality vegetarian diet.

OMEGA-9 FATS

The *Journal of the National Cancer Institute* has reported that a serving of olive oil a day lowered the risk of breast cancer by 25 percent in Greek women. The study's author, Harvard's Dr. Dimitrios Trichopoulos, believes that American women might expect at least a 50 percent reduction in breast cancer by this substitution. Why? First, even those Greek women eating the least amount of olive oil consumed more than virtually any American women. Second, women in Mediterranean countries already have a 50 percent lower risk of breast cancer than American women, so the expectation is that American women may benefit even more if olive oil is substituted for dangerous fats found in vegetable oils and margarines. There are now four case-controlled studies from the Mediterranean showing a strong protective benefit of olive oil.

BREAST BENEFITS OF OLIVE OIL

As you eliminate omega-6 fatty acids from your diet, and add omega-9 fatty acids, your breast too will accumulate more omega-9 fatty acids, neutralizing the booster effect. As olive oil displaces starches in the diet of Mediterranean peoples, the risk of breast cancer actually decreases. Olive oil is also loaded with powerful antioxidants that can drop your oxidant load.

HOW TO USE OLIVE OIL

Olive oil should be used as a deliberate replacement for dangerous fats and refined carbohydrates. However, adding olive oil to these foods will do nothing more than make you fat. Dr. Scott Grundy of the famous Texas Health Sciences Center in Dallas has a simple recommendation. Just add two tablespoonfuls of olive oil to a healthy diet. You do this by adding it to a salad or vegetables. Or you can use it in cooking vegetables.

THE OLIVE OIL CONTROVERSY

You may say, hey, you said that fat may cause breast cancer — how can you recommend fat? You're right. Olive oil is a fat. If you eat enough of it, you will become fat. In fact Crete, the site of the healthiest diet in the world, has suffered a decline in the health of its citizens with the addition of more calories and more olive oil over the last several decades. The answer to your question is simple. If you are willing to eat a very high-quality vegetarian diet, without olive oil, that is your healthiest choice. However, if you currently eat a high-fat diet, you are far better off replacing omega-6 fats, transfats, and saturated fats with olive oil. If you currently eat a low-quality low-fat diet with lots of refined carbohydrates, you are far better off replacing those carbohydrates with olive oil.

OTHER MONOUNSATURATED FATS

Alicja Wolk, Ph.D., from the Karolinska Institute in Stockholm, Sweden, studied 61,471 women between the ages of 40 and 76 from 1987 to 1990. In the January 12, 1998, *Archives of Internal Medicine*, Dr. Wolk reported that monounsaturated fat reduced the risk of breast cancer by 45 percent. The study credited canola as well as olive oil. To date, the bulk of the world literature links the use of olive oil to less breast cancer. That's why most experts continue to recommend olive oil over other monounsaturated fats.

Recommendation

Include two tablespoonfuls of olive oil a day on salads or in cooking.

OMEGA-3 FATS

The one quick step you can take to cut your risk of breast cancer is to consume omega-3 fatty acids every day. Omega-3 fatty acids cut the estrogen booster effect more powerfully than any other food. Scientists first observed the protective effect of omega-3 fatty acids in Greenland Eskimo women, who appeared to have *no* breast cancer. These women have a diet with one of the highest concentrations of omega-3s on earth. When they went to the lab, scientists found that, sure enough, omega-3s cause human breast cancers to decrease in size in both test tubes and animals. They even prevented metastases to the lungs in mice. A French study showed the same phenomenon in humans. Women with the lowest amounts of an omega-3 fat in the tissue surrounding their tumors were five times as likely to develop metastatic disease.

BREAST BENEFITS OF OMEGA-3

Fish oils can change the microenvironment of the breast in an astoundingly short, three-month period, quickly blunting the booster effect. By taking 10 grams of fish oils a day, breast cancer survivors at UCLA tripled the amount of omega-3 fatty acids in their breasts. The body stores such an enormous amount of omega-6 fats that it would take at least three years to wash them out of your system. During those three years, you want to protect yourself with omega-3 fatty acids, which will strongly counteract them. Clinical trials are now under way in breast cancer survivors at UCLA based on a wealth of human observation and animal and test-tube data. Women in these trials have tripled the amount of omega-3 fats in their breasts.

Safety

As powerful as the effects of omega-3 fatty acids are, it's also critical to look at them for their safety. At very high doses, omega-3 fatty acids cause bleeding — even bleeding into the brain. You may say, gosh, that's a hell of a risk to take to prevent cancer. The good news is that that dose is many times what you need to take. Thousands of American women at high risk or who are breast cancer survivors now take omega-3s at their doctor's recommendation. Doctors from Sloan-Kettering to UCLA feel comfortable prescribing omega-3s for their patients. If you take blood thinners or have clotting problems, be sure to have your blood-clotting factors measured if you and your doctor opt to try this strategy.

There are two other side effects, diarrhea and smell. Diarrhea affects a minority of women. A good way to avoid this side effect is to go easy, by starting with just a gram a day. Fish oil does smell, if it is of poor quality. Buy high-quality oils and use them quickly to avoid the smell. The longer fish oil capsules sit, the quicker the fish smell and flavor comes back, even if it's been steam-stripped.

Dose

Patients in the UCLA trial consumed 10 grams of fish oil per day, which translates into 10 fish oil capsules daily. These capsules were taken in a divided dose three times a day: breakfast 3, lunch 3, and dinner 4. The brand used at UCLA is Nature Made vitamins (ProEPA, Mission Hills, CA). Dr. John Glaspy determined that at the 10-gram dose there was no increased tendency to bleed. However, if you have a bleeding disorder, or are taking aspirin or NSAID therapy (Motrin, Advil, ibuprofen) or an anticoagulant, you can ask your doctor to perform a bleeding test called a PTT (partial thromboplastin time) to be certain that fish oils don't increase your risk of bleeding. In one major cancer center, patients were accidentally given a large overdose. While there was no bleeding, women did rapidly gain weight and facial hair. The not-so-funny joke was that they had begun to look like the Eskimo women who gave doctors the idea in the first place. Since 10 grams works and works quickly, there is no need for a higher dose. UCLA adds 800 IU of vitamin E a day to prevent oxidation of the fish oil. Since a recent study showed vitamin E may increase the risk of breast cancer, you'll want to ask your doctor if adding vitamin E to fish oil makes sense. Since capsules are much more palatable than fish oil in liquid form, virtually all clinical trials opt for capsules.

Fish oils are now being recommended as a part of any program of healthy living. If you and your doctor decide against fish oil capsules as part of your breast cancer prevention program, you should still consider ingesting the generally recommended 1- to 2-gram-a-day dose in the foods that you eat. While the U.S. government has not made a recommendation on fish oil ingestion, England has. The British Nutrition Foundation recommends 1.25 grams a day. Practically speaking, it's difficult to get much more than 2 grams a day of fish oils without the use of supplements.

Source

The American Health Foundation, Memorial Sloan-Kettering Cancer Center, and UCLA plus most major medical centers conducting clinical trials are dispensing omega-3 fatty acids in pill form in order to determine exactly how much omega-3 women have consumed. Clearly, omega-3 from fish would be vastly preferable; it is better absorbed, and it comes with many other nutrients. However, fish fat can concentrate chemical estrogens. The chapter "Step 8: Avoid Chemical Estrogens" tells you which fish are safe and which are not. At home we like to alternate between supplements and fish. The days we have a big piece of salmon for lunch, we'll skip the fish oil capsule.

CONSUMER'S GUIDE TO SUPPLEMENTS

For those who cannot or will not eat fish or for those concerned about the heavy metals and pesticides contained in fish, supplements are the only way to go. For women at high risk of breast cancer, this is the fastest, most effective way of changing breast fat. However, most top researchers in the field feel that women should take large amounts of fish oil for significant periods only under the confines of a research study or careful clinical observation.

Contaminants

Fish oils are so highly processed that it would probably be impossible to find any measurable amounts of contaminants, say experts assembled by the Food and Nutrition Board of the Institute of Medicine of the National Academy of Sciences. Heavy metals don't accumulate in fish oil because the processing techniques take it out. Steam-stripping removes pesticides, PCBs, and heavy metals. Fish oils that taste very "fishy" may not be steam-stripped. Look for "molecularly distilled" fish oils for the cleanest product.

REAL FISH

New data shows almost nonexistent levels of pesticide or heavy metal contamination in fish. These levels have dramatically dropped in species used for obtaining omega-3 oils, according to the U.S. Department of Fisheries. There are no good alternative sources of information to confirm or deny this level of safety. Several meals a week of fish is a good recommendation.

The table on pages 88–90 lays out the total amount of omega-3 fatty acids in various fish and fish oils. Look for the omega-3 fatty acids EPA and DHA. They stand for eicosapentaenoic acid and docosahexaenoic acid. They are the most critically important omega-3 fatty acids found in fish. The table lists the amount of EPA and DHA plus their combined total. (New food labeling that will include omega-3 content is being considered.) Fish oils are shown at the top for comparison. For the fish richest in fish oil, 100 grams of fish flesh will contain 2 grams of fish oil (100 grams is slightly less than a quarter of a pound). As you can see, to consume 10 grams of fish oil is the equivalent of eating a pound and a quarter of fish a day! That's a pretty remarkable amount. Practically speaking, you can get the first 2 grams by eating fish; any more and you're stuck with fish oil capsules.

A special note on tuna: Oil-packed tuna usually employs omega-6 vegetable oil, really defeating the purpose of eating the fish in the first place. Do shop for water-packed tuna and look to be sure that it has a high fish oil content.

Cod liver oil has high amounts of vitamins A and D. This on its own is a good thing, but to eat 10 grams a day of fish oils might mean taking an overdose of vitamins A and D. The oil-based vitamins A and D accumulate in the body and don't flush out, so you can accumulate toxic amounts.

OMEGA-3 FATTY ACIDS IN FISH AND FISH OILS

Fish Oils/Fish	Omega-3 Fatty Acids		Total Fish Oil (per 100 grams)
	EPA	DHA	
MaxEPATM, concentrated fish body oils	17.8	11.6	29.4
Menhaden oil	12.7	7.9	20.6
Salmon oil	8.8	11.1	19.9
Cod liver oil	9.0	9.5	18.5
Herring oil	7.1	4.3	11.4
Atlantic mackerel	0.9	1.6	2.5
King mackerel	1	1.2	2.2
Muroaji scad	0.5	1.5	2.0
Chub mackerel	0.9	1	1.9
Spiny dogfish	0.7	1.2	1.9
Japanese horse mackerel	0.5	1.3	1.8
Pacific herring	1.0	0.7	1.7
Atlantic herring	0.7	0.9	1.6
Lake trout	0.5	1.1	1.6
Bluefin tuna	0.4	1.2	1.6
Atlantic sturgeon	1.0	0.5	1.5
Sablefish	0.7	0.7	1.4
Chinook salmon	0.8	0.6	1.4
European anchovy	0.5	0.9	1.4
Albacore tuna	0.3	1.0	1.3

Omega-3 Fats

Fish Oils/Fish	Omega-3 Fatty Acids		Total Fish Oil (per 100 grams)
	EPA	DHA	
Lake whitefish	0.3	1.0	1.3
Saury	0.5	0.8	1.3
European sole	0.5	0.8	1.3
Sprat	0.5	0.8	1.3
Atlantic salmon	0.3	0.9	1.2
Round herring	0.4	0.8	1.2
Sockeye salmon	0.5	0.7	1.2
Bluefish	0.4	0.8	1.2
Unspecified mullet	0.5	0.6	1.1
Chum salmon	0.4	0.6	1.0
Coho salmon	0.3	0.5	0.8
Pink salmon	0.4	0.6	1.0
Unspecified conch	0.6	0.4	1.0
Greenland halibut	0.5	0.4	0.9
Striped bass	0.2	0.6	0.8
Rainbow smelt	0.3	0.4	0.7
Rockfish	0.3	0.4	0.7
Pompano	0.2	0.4	0.6
Pacific oyster	0.4	0.2	0.6
Horse mackerel	0.3	0.3	0.6
Swordfish	0.1	0.5	0.6
Arctic char trout	0.1	0.5	0.6
Atlantic wolffish	0.3	0.3	0.6
Common periwinkle	0.5	0	0.5

Fish Oils/Fish	Omega-3 Fatty Acids		Total Fish Oil (per 100 grams)
	EPA	DHA	
Freshwater drum	0.2	0.3	0.5
Silver hake	0.2	0.3	0.5
Striped mullet	0.3	0.2	0.5
Rainbow trout	0.1	0.4	0.5
European oyster	0.3	0.2	0.5
Pacific hake	0.2	0.3	0.5
Pollock	0.1	0.4	0.5
Canary rockfish	0.2	0.3	0.5
Unspecified rockfish	0.2	0.3	0.5
Unspecified shark	0	0.5	0.5
Unspecified tuna	0.1	0.4	0.5
Japanese (kuruma) prawn	0.3	0.2	0.5
Northern shrimp	0.3	0.2	0.5
Blue mussel	0.2	0.3	0.5
Brook trout	0.2	0.2	0.4
Brown bullhead catfish	0.2	0.2	0.4
Cisco	0.1	0.3	0.4
Pacific halibut	0.1	0.3	0.4
Carp	0.2	0.1	0.3
Sweet smelt	0.2	0.1	0.3
European eel	0.1	0.1	0.2

U.S. Department of Agriculture

Other Benefits

Omega-3s are increasingly being found to be powerful super-nutrients for a variety of diseases from rheumatoid arthritis and multiple sclerosis to heart disease. In fact, omega-3s are being promoted as the heart-healthiest fat. Eating lots of fish is even better than a vegetarian diet for reducing levels of certain blood fats that increase the risk of heart attack.

Analysis

Fish oils are the fastest and most effective way of changing breast fats. Aggressive studies are under way to prove they can lower the risk of cancer in human beings. Committing to a year or two of use while waiting to see how clinical trials develop should prove a low-risk proposition.

Recommendation

Using supplements or safe fish sources, take 10 grams of fish oil a day if you are at high breast cancer risk, and 2 grams a day if you are at lower risk.

STEP 3: MAKE

GOOD ESTROGENS

Only one kind of vegetable interferes with the estrogen pathway and that is a cruciferous vegetable. These get their name from the crosslike stem they all have in common, from broccoli to cauliflower. European women who ate more cabbage had a lower breast cancer death rate. Cruciferous vegetables decreased the risk by 40 percent in a Wisconsin study. How do they work? Their secret ingredient is called indole-3 carbinol, which channels the breakdown products of estrogen into far more "good" estrogen (2-hydroxyestrone) than "bad" estrogen (16-alpha-hydroxyestrone). As with the good and bad cholesterol in your blood, you can increase and decrease the amount of either form of estrogen. The *Journal of the National Cancer Institute* reported that the "bad" estrogen may be a major factor in breast cancer development in Finnish women, since it permanently binds to the estrogen receptor — sort of like pressing a car horn and finding it's stuck. All other estrogens attach briefly and then are released. Strang Cancer Prevention

Center's Dr. Jack Fishman believes bad estrogen could be a very big part of the whole picture. Women with breast cancer have almost twice as much bad estrogen as those without. Bad estrogen also causes mutations in breast cells. Another "bad" estrogen (4 hydroxy) may directly damage DNA, reports Dr. Ercole Cavaliere of the Eppley Institute for Research in Cancer at the University of Nebraska Medical Center.

BREAST BENEFITS
OF CRUCIFEROUS VEGETABLES

The active ingredient in cruciferous vegetables, indole-3 carbinol, diverts estrogen into more "good" estrogens. Indole-3 carbinol can double the amount of good estrogen while decreasing the bad, as reported in a study in the *Journal of the National Cancer Institute*. My friend Jon Michnovicz, M.D., of the Strang Cancer Prevention Center calls this a detoxifying pathway. A University of California at Berkeley study shows that the indole-3 carbinol from broccoli halts the growth of breast cancer cells by turning off a key enzyme important for the cells' growth cycle.

KINDS OF VEGETABLES CONTAINING
INDOLE-3 CARBINOL

Bitter cress	Cabbage
Bok choy	Cauliflower
Broccoli	Collard
Brussels sprouts	Horseradish

Kale	Savoy cabbage
Mustard seed	Super broccoli
Radishes	Turnip
Rutabaga	Watercress

Supertasters

Don't like cruciferous vegetables? Little wonder. You are what scientists call a "supertaster," a person who finds these vegetables taste unusually bitter. Researchers believe that you are at a genetic disadvantage because you won't eat the vegetables that have the most powerful cancer-fighting effect. I've got to admit I'm one. I've never liked these vegetables and neither does my family. I do like fresh broccoli, not the limp steamed kind. Coleslaw may be the most palatable choice of cruciferous vegetable — if made with the right low-fat dressing.

CONSUMER TIPS

The active ingredient, indole-3 carbinol, can be deactivated by heat. For that reason you'll want to avoid badly wilted cruciferous vegetables. Lightly steaming or stir-frying them can maintain the active ingredient.

Dose

Pioneers Leon Bradlow and Jack Fishman conducted a "dosing" study of indole-3 carbinol and found no beneficial effect until volunteers ingested 300 milligrams a day. The fly in the ointment is that you'd have to eat an enormous amount of cruciferous vegetables to ingest those 300 milligrams, the equivalent of two heads of cabbage. One published study showed that 500 milligrams created a pronounced shift toward the good estrogen — that's approximately *fifty* times what the average American currently eats. Japanese and Chinese women who eat large amounts of cruciferous vegetables consume only 100 milligrams of I3C per day. The bottom line is that its incredibly difficult to get 300 milligrams a day from eating cruciferous vegetables. The Strang lab recommends eating these vegetables for the indole-3 carbinol and for their fiber, vitamin, and antioxidant properties — but to get the full effect, you'll need to supplement. Capsules are the best way to ensure that you're getting enough indole-3 carbinol, and they're readily available in health food stores. Don't take antacids when taking capsules or eating cruciferous vegetables because they interfere with absorption; 300 to 500 milligrams a day will increase the production of food estrogens.

Recommendation

Eat two or more servings of cruciferous vegetables a day. Consider, with your physician, taking 500 milligrams of indole-3 carbinol as a supplement if you are at high risk.

STEP 4:

LOWER INSULIN

Not long ago exciting, first-ever evidence finally linked insulin to breast cancer. In her striking breakthrough research, Dr. Pamela Goodwin, from the University of Toronto, found one of the highest risks in this book, a 283 percent increased risk of breast cancer in women with high insulin levels. She studied 99 premenopausal women who were just diagnosed with node-negative breast cancer and 99 age-matched women who were biopsied but didn't have cancer. What is so striking about this study is that many of these women were quite lean. This is one of the first clues as to why lean premenopausal women may be at increased risk for breast cancer. Another group, out of St. Thomas Hospital in London, also postulates that the high insulin that results from high animal fat intake and weight gain after the age of thirty could contribute to the increase in post-menopausal breast cancer. "Case-control studies have shown that high insulin and abdominal obesity are risk markers for postmenopausal breast cancer. Too much insulin may also stimulate growth activity in existing breast cancer."

Most of us know insulin as the hormone that regulates blood sugar levels. However, it has a far more nefarious role. Insulin acts as a growth factor for cancer development. Here's how. There are insulin receptors on the surfaces of breast cells just like there are estrogen receptors. Insulin enhances the likelihood that cells become cancerous by attaching to these receptors. Cancer cells also have insulin receptors. When insulin attaches to the receptor, it turns it on, leading to cancer growth.

Clearly a high insulin level provides much more stimulation for the breast cell to change, grow, or divide. How high that insulin level rises is directly related to your diet.

HOW TO DETERMINE YOUR INSULIN LEVEL

The next time you have blood work, ask your doctor to include an insulin level. It's available at most commercial labs. The insulin level is measured after an overnight fast and can range from 79, an excellent value, to 190, considered very high. As you'd expect, insulin levels are high in women with excess body fat, especially if that fat is carried above the waist.

A close friend of my wife and mine was diagnosed with breast cancer at age 39. She is quite lean and wondered how it was possible for her to contract breast cancer if she wasn't overweight. The most interesting contributing factor that's come forward is a high insulin level. Surprisingly, insulin levels are highest in the thinnest women. Women who eat a high-refined-flour, low-fiber diet, even if it is low in fat, are especially apt to run high insulin levels.

HOW TO LOWER YOUR INSULIN LEVEL

If your blood sugar and insulin levels are elevated, you may have Type II diabetes. This illness can result in severe complications, from blindness and heart disease to loss of a kidney or limb. You will want to consult with an endocrinologist who specializes in diabetes to plan your treatment. A cornerstone of the treatment of anyone with high insulin should be to lower glucose load. Whether you have diabetes or simply have an insulin level high enough to increase your risk of breast cancer, the following steps to lower your insulin level will be extremely useful.

Avoid Saturated Fats

Saturated fats increase insulin resistance. Insulin resistance simply means that your body does not react to normal amounts of insulin and admits sugar into cells. This causes your body to make much higher levels of insulin to compensate, thus contributing to weight gain and cancer risk. Key saturated fats are found in whole dairy products and fatty red meats.

Decrease Upper Body Obesity

Decreasing obesity leads to lowered insulin resistance and decreased production of insulin.

Exercise

Regular physical activity has long been shown to decrease insulin requirements. It does so by allowing sugar into muscle cells lacking insulin so that the body does not have to make as much.

Decrease Glucose Load

Given the critical importance of glucose load to weight loss and lowering insulin levels, the following chapter is devoted to showing you how to decrease glucose load.

Note: The increased risk of breast cancer linked to insulin does not apply to Type I diabetics who make no insulin of their own. It does apply to Type II diabetics who make too much insulin to compensate for insulin resistance.

Recommendation

To lower your insulin level, avoid saturated fats and reduce your glucose load.

STEP 5:

DROP GLUCOSE

OVERLOAD

In my last book, *Dr. Bob Arnot's Revolutionary Weight Control Program,* I called glucose load the premier concept in nutrition today, the most effective way of becoming lean and controlling your weight. Since publication of that book, dozens of new articles have appeared in the scientific literature supporting the concept and demonstrating the links between high load and other diseases, from heart disease to childhood obesity. Now it is linked to breast cancer. A high-starch diet predicted breast cancer in an Italian population by a substantial 40 percent.

First let's look at what we mean by the term "glucose load." As I reported in *Revolutionary Weight Control,* from hard candy to complex carbohydrates, ultimately most carbohydrates are broken down into glucose. Glucose load is a measure of the total amount of glucose that passes through the bloodstream in a day. The more glucose jammed into the bloodstream the higher the glucose load. After a large meal, that "load" can reach significant levels and signal the body to produce large amounts of insulin. Now, many of us falsely believe that it's only candy bars, ice cream, sugary sodas, and other sweets that affect glucose levels. Most weight-conscious women believe that they successfully avoid these sugary foods, and that's the trap. They eat, instead, hundreds of foods that rapidly convert into glucose. The most surprising are some highly promoted "complex carbohydrates." White flour products, from pasta and cereal to bagels and breads, all earn the title "complex carbos." Many are even labeled "low-fat" foods. Though these carbohydrates are indeed complex because they are made up of enormous sugar molecules instead of tiny "simple" sugars, these quickly break down into glucose, many faster than table sugar itself. When you sum up the total of all the glucose produced by a day's worth of carbohydrates, you arrive at what researchers call your total glucose load. To determine your glucose load, you first need to know how much each individual food will raise your blood sugar. Here's how that is determined.

DETERMINING THE GLUCOSE CONTENT OF INDIVIDUAL FOODS

After you eat a food on an empty stomach, your blood sugar is measured at regular intervals until a peak level is detected. Dr. David Jenkins of the University of Toronto and other researchers made this measurement for hundreds of foods. Each carbohydrate was assigned a glucose value on a scale that ranges from a low of 0 to a high of over 100. (Researchers use the term "glycemic index," while nutrition aficionados use the abbreviation "GI.") Carbohydrates low on the index, such as beans, generate a very small rise in blood sugar after they are eaten. That puts an insignificant "load" on your system. Foods with a high glycemic index, from instant mashed potatoes and white bread, Twinkies, and muffins to bagels, are digested very quickly, giving rise to high blood sugars. Since these high-glycemic-index foods are basically glucose bombs, the more of these foods in your diet the higher your blood sugar.

Most nutrition-conscious consumers know to avoid foods with a high glycemic index, but where virtually all of us go wrong is with too many medium-glycemic-index foods such as rice, pasta, potatoes, and white flour products. These carbohydrates, comprising thousands of glucose molecules strung together, enter your body like a Trojan horse. Since they don't taste sweet or look sweet, we eat tons of them — falsely believing that they are healthy for us. But once your digestive tract strips their disguise by breaking them apart, millions of glucose molecules flow freely into your bloodstream like water through a broken dike. To calculate glucose load, add up the individual glycemic index of each carbohydrate you eat. Here's an example:

These four "complex carbohydrates," each of which has an astoundingly high glycemic index, have a sky-high glucose load, adding up to a total of 351.

French baguette	95
Instant rice	87

Baked potato	85
Corn flakes	84
TOTAL	351

However, what troubles the nation's leading nutritionists is that you need not have foods with an outrageously high glycemic index to have a high glucose load. Foods with a moderate glycemic index, like white rice or pasta, can give you a sky-high glucose load if you eat more than several servings a day. While individual foods that cause large rises in blood sugar are said to have a high glycemic index, an entire meal built on foods with a high or even medium glycemic index is said to have a high glucose load. Now let's look at the effect of five moderate-glycemic-index foods on glucose load.

Pizza with cheese	60
White potato	56
White pita bread	57
Durum spaghetti	55
Tortellini with cheese	50
TOTAL	278

That glucose load still adds up to a whopping 278.

HOW GLUCOSE OVERLOAD MAKES YOU FAT

Excess insulin is the most likely reason that you are overweight and the biggest reason that those extra pounds will kill you. Insulin is the trigger that switches your body's weight-gaining functions into high gear and is the hormone most responsible for the ballooning of America. How? Too much insulin jam-packs fat cells with fats, slams the door, and throws away the key. What's the link between glucose load and insulin? The higher your glucose load, the higher your insulin level because it is glucose load that drives insulin. Insulin is up to thirty times more effective at moving extra calories into fat than into muscle, making it an effective super stuffer of fat cells. The more fat you eat the further those floodgates swing open. That's why the combination of fat and high glycemic index is so incredibly fattening.

BREAST BENEFITS OF A LOW GLUCOSE LOAD

A low glucose load decreases insulin levels, hunger, and upper body fat. A low glucose load also decreases the amount of triglycerides in the blood. A recent study demonstrates that women with elevated triglyceride levels had an increased risk of breast cancer.

HOW TO DROP GLUCOSE LOAD

Avoid Foods with a High Glycemic Index

These foods cause the largest increase in your blood sugar level. You'll find some real surprises on this list such as bagels, hamburger buns, instant rice, and macaroni with cheese. The higher the number in the table on pages 105–7, the higher your blood sugar will rise after you eat them! If you really love these foods, mix them with extremely low GI foods — once you've lost the weight you want to. An example would be low-GI soybeans mixed with high-GI rice, which averages out to a moderate glucose load.

HIGH-GLYCEMIC-INDEX FOODS

Food	Glycemic Index
Hamburger bun	61
Ice cream	61
New potato	62
Semolina	64
Shortbread	64
Raisins	64
Macaroni and cheese, boxed	64
Rye flour	65
Couscous	65
High-fiber crisp rye bread	65
Sucrose	65
Cream of Wheat (cereal)	66
Life (cereal)	66
Muesli (cereal)	66
Pineapple	66
Angel food cake	67
Croissant	67
Grape-Nuts (cereal)	67

Food	Glycemic Index
Puffed Wheat (cereal)	67
Stoned Wheat Thins	67
Soft drink, Fanta	68
Cornmeal maize	68
Mars Bar	68
English muffin	69
Wheat bread, gluten-free	69
Shredded Wheat (cereal)	69
Melba toast	70
Wheat biscuits	70
Potato, white, mashed	70
Life Savers	70
Fruit, dried	70
Golden Grahams (crackers)	71
Millet	71
Carrot	71
Bagel, white	72
Water crackers	72
Watermelon	72
Popcorn	72
Kaiser rolls	73
Potato, boiled, mashed	73
Corn chips	73
Honey	73
Bread stuffing	74
Cheerios (cereal)	74
French fries	75

Food	Glycemic Index
Pumpkin	75
Donut	76
Waffle	76
Cocoa Puffs (cereal)	77
Vanilla wafers	77
Broad beans	79
Grape-Nuts Flakes (cereal)	80
Jelly beans	80
Rice Krispies (cereal)	82
Rice cake	82
Corn Chex (cereal)	83
Potato, instant mashed	83
Corn flakes (cereal)	84
Potato, baked	85
Crispix (cereal)	87
Rice, instant	87
Rice, white, low amylose	88
Rice Chex (cereal)	89
Cactus jam	91
Rice pasta, brown	92
French baguette	95
Rockmelon	95
Parsnip	97
Glucose tablets	102
Maltose	105
Tofu frozen dessert, nondairy	115

Table adapted with permission from the American Journal of Clinical Nutrition 62 *(1995): 871–935.*

An excess of glucose makes most people sleepier than they otherwise would be, leading them to eat even more in an attempt to increase energy.

Avoid Most Moderate-Glycemic-Index Foods

If you are really trying to lose weight, eliminate these foods as well. The real surprise is how much medium-glycemic-index foods add to the glucose load. They appear to be safe and conventional, but eaten in even moderate quantities they will make you fat. The higher the foods' glycemic index, the higher your blood sugar will be after eating them. A diet full of them will keep you hungry. Just think of how hungry you are after a meal of Chinese takeout, which is heavy on rice and noodles. The food literally washes through your system too fast to keep you satisfied for long.

MODERATE-GLYCEMIC-INDEX FOODS

Food	Glycemic Index
Capellini	45
Macaroni, boiled 5 minutes	45
Romano beans	46
Linguine, thick durum	46
Lactose	46
Fruit loaf, wheat with dried fruit	47
Instant noodles	47
Bulgur	48
Baked beans	48

Step 5: Drop Glucose Overload

Food	Glycemic Index
Green peas	48
Corn, high amylose	49
Chocolate	49
Rye kernel	50
Ice cream, low fat	50
Tortellini, cheese	50
Yam	51
Kiwifruit	52
Banana	53
Special K (cereal)	54
Buckwheat	54
Sweet potato	54
Potato chips	54
Fruit cocktail, canned	55
Mango	55
Spaghetti, durum	55
Sweet corn	55
Potato, white	56
Pita, white	57
Orange juice	57
Bran Chex (cereal)	58
Peach, canned, heavy syrup	58
Rice vermicelli	58
Blueberry	59
Rice, white, high amylose	59
Pizza, cheese	60

Table adapted with permission from the American Journal of Clinical Nutrition 62 (1995):871–935.

Substitute Low-Glycemic-Index Foods for All Other Carbos

Low-glycemic-index foods drop your insulin level. The Pritikin Longevity Center in Santa Monica, California, reports a fall in the average fasting insulin of 25 to 30 percent for those individuals eating carbohydrates in their "very unrefined state." You may literally eat all the low-GI carbos you want because they are so filling and have such a small effect on glucose load. Examples are beans, cruciferous vegetables, and high-fiber, low-sugar cereals.

LOW-GLYCEMIC-INDEX FOODS

Food	Glycemic Index
Nopales, prickly pear cactus	7
Yogurt, lowfat, unsweetened, plain	14
Acorns, stewed with venison	16
Soybeans	18
Rice bran	19
Cherries	22
Peas, dried	22
Plum	24
Barley	25
Grapefruit	25
Mesquite cake	25
Kidney beans	27
Peach, fresh	28
Beans, dried	29

Step 5: Drop Glucose Overload

Food	Glycemic Index
Lentils	29
Yellow tepary bean broth	29
Green beans	30
Black beans	30
Apricot, dried	31
Butter beans	31
Skim milk	32
Lima beans, baby, frozen	32
Split peas, yellow, boiled	32
Chickpeas	33
Rye rice	34
Apple	36
Pear	36
Spaghetti, whole wheat	37
Haricot (navy) beans	38
Star pastina, boiled 5 minutes	38
Tomato	38
Tortilla	38
Brown beans	38
Pinto beans	39
Corn hominy	40
All-Bran (cereal)	42
Black-eyed peas	42
Grapes	43
Orange	43
Spirali, durum	43
Mixed grain	45

Table adapted with permission from the American Journal of Clinical Nutrition 62 *(1995):871–935.*

Eat More Protein

When a meal is stripped of carbohydrate and only the protein remains, insulin levels rise very little. Protein also helps to kill hunger and energize the brain while keeping insulin levels low. Protein is a great way to displace junk carbohydrates from your diet. By replacing carbohydrate in a meal with protein you decrease your glucose load. The mark to aim for is 15 to 20 percent protein. Dean Ornish's program uses a higher protein intake to decrease triglycerides, which are also a risk factor. If you're incorporating soy into your program, you'll easily hit that mark. The danger of protein is only if you are on a very high-calorie diet and eating massive amounts.

Eat More Soluble Fiber

The higher your fiber intake, the lower your risk of running a high insulin level. Soluble fiber forms a gummy gel that lines the intestine and slows absorption, blunting the uptake of glucose and decreasing the insulin response. The following chapter includes a complete list of soluble fibers.

Recommendation

Avoid all foods with high and medium glycemic indexes until you have lowered your body weight to where you would like to be. Then, you may want to consider adding several medium-glycemic-index foods a day (if you really miss them!).

STEP 6:

INCREASE FIBER

Fiber may be the most underrated of all breast cancer preventive nutrients. Yet at major cancer centers such as Memorial Sloan-Kettering, it is finally getting its due. Moishe Shike, director of clinical nutrition, says "Absolutely, I think fiber is so important."

BREAST BENEFITS OF FIBER

There's little wonder why fiber is such a powerful preventive agent. Fiber interrupts most steps of the estrogen pathway to decrease the blood level of an estrogen called estrone sulfate by a powerful 36 percent. That translates into a 54 percent decrease in cancer risk for women on a high-fiber diet. David Rose reports in the journal *Nutrition* that "supplementing the diet with wheat bran to achieve a high fiber intake causes a significant reduction in . . . serum estrone and estradiol concentration of premenopausal women." Why? Fiber builds more estrogen carriers, traps estrogen in the bowel so it can't be re-circulated, decreases glucose load, cuts hunger, and speeds weight loss. Few Americans benefit from fiber because our diet is notoriously low in fiber by world standards. The lack of fiber allows free estrogen to soar.

Dose

Most studies don't show much of a relation between fiber and breast cancer, simply because most people consume so little fiber, an average of roughly 12 grams per day. Twenty grams of wheat bran alone significantly decreases estrogen levels. Sloan-Kettering recommends at least 25 to 30 grams for its breast cancer patients. I personally recommend 30 to 50 grams of fiber.

CONSUMER'S GUIDE TO FIBER

You will be quite surprised that most foods, even those famous for fiber, have vanishingly little fiber in them. This guide will help you select the foods that are highest in fiber. In choosing, keep in mind that there are two different kinds of fiber, insoluble and soluble. Here's how they stack up.

Insoluble fiber is best for binding estrogen in the bowel. The ingredient that binds estrogen most tightly is cellulose. Wheat bran is an excellent source of cellulose. The table on pages 115–17 lists the foods highest in insoluble fiber. When I look at the nutritional label on a package, I like to see at least 5 grams of fiber with less than 5 grams of sugar per serving.

HIGH-INSOLUBLE-FIBER FOODS

Food (100-gram portion)	*Insoluble Fiber (grams)*
CEREALS	
All Bran with Extra Fiber, Kellogg	46.20
Fiber One, General Mills	39.40
All Bran, Kellogg	25.70
Bran Flakes, Post	13.80
Raisin Bran, Post or Kellogg	11.10
Shredded Wheat, Post	10.90
GRAINS	
Corn bran, uncooked	80.40
Wheat bran	37.60
Wheat germ	14.30
Popcorn, popped	10.80
Flour, whole wheat	9.10
Flour, rye	9.00
Barley, pearl, uncooked	8.40
Spaghetti, whole wheat, uncooked	7.80
Macaroni, whole wheat, uncooked	6.90
Cornmeal, blue	6.90
Oatmeal, uncooked	4.60
Flour, oat	4.00

Food (100-gram portion)	Insoluble Fiber (grams)

BREADS AND CRACKERS

Crackers, snack, whole wheat	9.10
Melba toast, wheat	7.10
Rye bread (German)	6.80
Pumpernickel bread	4.50

FRUITS

Peaches, dried	4.20
Figs, dried	4.20
Apricots, dried	3.50
Prunes, dried	2.80

VEGETABLES

Okra, fresh, trimmed pods	4.40
Turnip, cooked	3.90
Brussels sprouts, fresh	2.70
Parsley, fresh	2.60
Brussels sprouts, cooked	2.40
Parsnip, cooked	1.90
Cabbage, winter, savoy, fresh	1.80
Celeriac, fresh	1.60

LEGUMES

White beans, Great Northern, dried, uncooked	13.30
Pinto beans, dried, uncooked	11.90
Kidney beans, dark red, dried, uncooked	11.30
Butter beans, dried, uncooked	10.60
Soybeans, dried, uncooked	10.50

Food (100-gram portion)	Insoluble Fiber (grams)
Lentils, dried, uncooked	10.30
Chickpeas, dried, uncooked	8.50
Mung beans, dried, uncooked	8.20
Split beans, dried, uncooked	5.10
Pinto beans, dried, cooked	4.70
Navy beans, dried, cooked	4.70
Kidney beans, dark red, dried, cooked	4.60
Butter beans, dried, cooked	4.40
Black beans, cooked	4.30
Pork and beans with sauce, cooked	2.20

NUTS AND SEEDS

Coconut, dried	14.90
Almonds	7.70
Coconut, fresh	7.70
Sesame seeds	7.20
Filberts (hazelnuts)	5.20
Peanuts, fresh	5.10
Peanuts, roasted	5.10
Sunflower seeds	4.00

BAKED GOODS

Oat Bran Graham Cookies, Health Valley	5.60
Oat Bran Fruit Jumbo Cookies, Health Valley	5.20
Oat Bran Animal Cookies, Health Valley	5.00

Adapted from Plant and Fiber in Foods, *2d ed. Courtesy of James W. Anderson, 1990, HCF Nutrition Research Foundation.*

ADDITIONAL BENEFITS

Heart Disease

For every extra gram you eat each day, your risk of heart disease decreases by 2 percent, as reported by the Harvard School of Public Health. My wife and I have found fiber to be the single most important factor in controlling our weight. By slowing digestion and making food "last longer," increased fiber causes hunger to drop rather dramatically. For instance, a key study looked at satiety with different kinds of breads. Where virtually fiber-free white bread could be eaten till the cows came home, higher-fiber whole wheat bread had a natural "brake" built into it. Study participants simply became full after a few slices — instead of working their way through an entire loaf. High-fiber foods are bulkier, have fewer calories, and take longer to eat, which gives your brain a chance to register your food intake before you overeat. Let's first look at the best "anti-hunger" fiber.

Soluble Fiber

This is the best fiber for controlling hunger, blood sugar, and cholesterol. It so successfully curbs hunger that it is justifiably called "the king of filler-uppers."

Soluble fiber is clearly the superior fiber, but you need not choose between the two types. Every food that contains 1 gram of soluble fiber usually contains another 3 grams of insoluble fiber. A high-fiber diet gives you excellent control over your blood sugar and insulin levels because the fiber holds sugars in the stomach so that they are released into the bloodstream far more slowly.

HIGH-SOLUBLE-FIBER FOODS

Food (100-gram portion)	Soluble Fiber (grams)

CEREALS

Oat bran, generic	7.6
Oat bran cereal, cold, Quaker	5.2
All-Bran, Kellogg	5.1
Oat bran cereal, hot, generic	4.8
Oatmeal Crisp, General Mills	4.5
Cheerios, General Mills	4.2
Complete Oat Bran Flakes, Kellogg	4.1
Complete Wheat Bran Flakes, Kellogg	3.5
Puffed Wheat, Quaker	3.4
All Bran with Extra Fiber, Kellogg	3.2
Grape-Nuts, Post	3.0
Fiber One, General Mills	3.0
Quaker Oatmeal Squares	2.9
Oat Bran Flakes, Health Valley	2.7
Nutri Grain, Kellogg	2.5
Wheaties, General Mills	2.4
Raisin Bran, Post or Kellogg	2.4
Total Whole Grain Wheat, General Mills	2.2
Shredded Wheat, Post	2.2

Food (100-gram portion)	Soluble Fiber (grams)
GRAINS	
Oat flour	5.5
Rye flour	3.9
Pearl barley, uncooked	3.4
Wheat bran	3.4
Wheat germ	3.2
Whole wheat flour	1.8
BREADS	
Pumpernickel bread	3.9
Rye bread	3.0
FRUITS	
Dried apricots	4.4
Dried figs	4.0
Dried prunes	3.8
Dried peaches	3.8
VEGETABLES	
Okra pods, fresh, trimmed	2.9
Parsley, fresh	2.8
Brussels sprouts, fresh, cooked	2.5
Turnip, cooked	2.2
Savoy winter cabbage, fresh	2.0
LEGUMES	
Kidney beans, dark red, dried, cooked	3.2
Cranberry beans, dried, cooked	3.1

Food (100-gram portion)	Soluble Fiber (grams)
Butter beans, dried, cooked	2.9
Black beans, cooked	2.8
Navy beans, dried, cooked	2.4
Pinto beans, dried, cooked	2.2
NUTS AND SEEDS	
Filberts (hazelnuts)	2.5
Sunflower seeds	2.1
BAKED GOODS	
Oat bran animal cookies	2.5
Oat bran fancy fruit muffin	2.4
Oat bran fruit jumbo cookies	2.4
Oat bran fruit and nut cookies	2.0

This table is reprinted with permission from the HCF Nutrition Research Foundations, Inc.

From a purely practical standpoint, you'll find beans and high-fiber breakfast cereals to be the most reasonable way to eat large quantities of soluble fiber. Otherwise you're faced with eating huge quantities of vegetables or grains. For instance, you would need 1,600 calories of Brussels sprouts to get 10 grams of soluble fiber. Contrast that to one cup of soybeans, which contains 10 grams of soluble fiber.

Start slowly! A cup of beans rich in soluble fiber can make you uncomfortably full for many hours; in fact you may still feel full 12 hours later. You may even feel guilty that you've eaten too much. What will surprise you is that you are far fuller on just 300 calories of beans than you ever would be on 1,500 calories of prime rib and potatoes. Soluble fibers are pulling water into the upper intestine, creating even more bulk and a greater sense of fullness. To avoid a sense of discomfort, begin by eating no more than a half of a cup of soluble-fiber foods per day. Increase your ration by one quarter cup every several days until you reach one and a half cups. If you've eaten what you think are lots of high-fiber foods and failed to get the effect that you've just read about, take a close look at the kind of fiber you've been eating. Most processed foods are notoriously poor in soluble fiber.

The other major concern is gas. In the first two weeks of a high-fiber diet, you will notice an increase in gas. However as the "good" gut bacteria win over the "bad," you'll find that it disappears.

Analysis

Fiber is a highly effective way of controlling weight and cholesterol level and of interfering with the estrogen pathway. Because of its overall health-promoting benefits there is no downside to fiber.

Recommendation

Eat 35 to 60 grams of fiber per day. If you're trying to control your hunger or weight, be sure 10 grams of that total is soluble fiber.

STEP 7:

LOWER OXIDATIVE

LOAD

Through most of this book we have looked at a highly targeted approach, how to intercept the critical estrogen pathway and achieve a substantial alteration in the pathway that fuels the growth and development of cancer. This chapter is quite different. It is aimed at blocking the initiation of cancer. Since we know so little about what pulls the trigger and converts a normal cell to a cancerous one, the approach is general, lowering oxidative load. The most effective way of lowering oxidative load is with the fruits and vegetables that are the most powerful *antiox-idants*. The great good news is that researchers have observed a 40 percent decrease in breast cancer for women who eat a diet rich in vegetables, even before fruit is added to the diet.

BREAST-PROTECTIVE EFFECTS
OF FRUITS AND VEGETABLES

A diet high in fruits and vegetables is the most powerful proactive step you can take to lower oxidant load. These foods also displace starches to cut glucose load.

Dose: So how much should you eat? If you really want to drop your oxidative load, nine servings of vegetables and fruit a day is the way to go. That's the maximum recommended by the National Cancer Institute. Most high fruit and vegetable interventions use a nine-a-day program. While that sounds like a lot, vegetables are the most nutrient-dense source of minerals, vitamins, and other key nutrients. You're also getting the greatest number of nutrients for the fewest number of calories. These foods are high in the fibers that fight hunger and will naturally displace fats and refined carbohydrates in your diet. With nine a day, blood levels of carotenoids can double in healthy people. Carotenoids are the pigments that give vegetables and fruits their colors such as green, yellow, and red. Carotenoids have strong antioxidant and anticancer qualities. Beta-carotene is the most popular example, with lutein, zeaxanthin, and lycopene quickly gaining widespread scientific respect as powerful antioxidants. Carotenoids take about six days to hit peak blood levels.

Intake of vegetables and fruits should be distributed throughout the day. Here's why. Oxidant load is reduced as soon as food is eaten and digested because the nutrients are absorbed into the blood. Carotenoids increase in blood right after meals. For example, there is a detectable increase in lycopene six hours after a meal of tomatoes, after which the level falls. Lycopene gives tomatoes their red color. Rats given a lycopene-enriched tomato formulation developed far fewer and much smaller breast cancers than rats without lycopene. New findings show that lycopene is most likely the carotenoid responsible for the protection against heart disease and cancer that had long been credited to beta-carotene. Lycopene is a much more powerful inhibitor of breast cancer growth than is beta-carotene. Curiously, lycopene is not well absorbed unless it has been cooked and concentrated. That makes tomato sauce, tomato paste, ketchup, and heated tomato juice the best sources. Vine-ripened tomatoes have the most lycopene.

Many women find that the easiest way of following such a diet is to become a vegetarian. In fact vegetarians have lower amounts of estrogen and less breast cancer — as evidenced by studies of Seventh-Day Adventists, who are strict vegetarians.

MEASURING OXIDATIVE LOAD

So you eat nine fruits and vegetables a day. Is it doing any good? Dr. Zora Djuric, Ph.D., a breast cancer specialist at Detroit's Barbara Ann Karmanos Cancer Institute, has developed an inventive, first-of-a-kind test for oxidative load. Are your genes being pummeled by a daily firestorm of oxidative damage? Dr. Djuric's test can tell you. She actually measures direct damage to DNA. Dr. Djuric has already been able to assess oxidative load in patients and determine the effect of diet. The surprise? The same diet has vastly different effects on different individuals. Five fruits and vegetables may be enough to quench the oxidative flame in some, while nine is too little in others. Within the next year this test may become available, allowing you to determine where your diet stands.

Do I believe that some foods are better than others? Absolutely! You will find charts here that display the most nutritious fruits and vegetables and special descriptions of those that have distinct effects.

VEGETABLES

The unique and invaluable table on page 127 shows the ability of vegetables to act as antioxidants. The actual values are expressed as ORAC, or "oxygen radical absorbence capacity." The oxygen radical is the substance that causes damage to genetic material. The ability of any antioxidant to soak up oxygen radicals is called absorbency. Despite all the hype, I was still surprised to see that garlic tops the list of foods able to absorb oxygen radicals. The more foods you eat from the top of this list the better. By coincidence, those vegetables that are best at making more good estrogen, from Brussels sprouts and broccoli to cabbage, are also great antioxidants. The best news is that palate-friendly vegetables like garlic, kale, onions, corn, and sweet potatoes are so high on the list.

Looking for an easy rule of thumb to accumulate all the vegetables you need? Dr. Zora Djuric urges women in her studies to eat a wide variety of fruits and vegetables to make

ANTIOXIDANT CAPACITY
OF SELECTED VEGETABLES

Vegetable	Antioxidant capacity
Garlic	19.4
Kale	17.7
Spinach	12.6
Brussels sprouts	9.8
Alfalfa sprouts	9.3
Broccoli flowerets	8.9
Beets	8.4
Red bell pepper	7.1
Onion	4.5
Corn	4.0
Eggplant	3.9
Cauliflower	3.8
Potato	3.1
Sweet potato	3.0
Cabbage	3.0
Leaf lettuce	2.6
Carrot	2.1
String bean	2.0
Yellow squash	1.5
Iceberg lettuce	1.2
Celery	0.6
Cucumber	0.5

Table adapted from Journal of Agricultural and Food Chemistry *44 (1996): 3426–3431.*

sure they get a lot of different antioxidants. She recommends five servings for daily intake, as follows:

- 1 red vegetable
- 1 orange vegetable
- 1 dark green vegetable
- 2 other vegetables

Serving size:
- ½ cup of cooked vegetables, or
- 1 cup raw leafy vegetables

FRUITS

If you're not in love with vegetables, the good news is that many fruits rival even the best vegetables at dropping your oxidative load.

ANTIOXIDANT CAPACITY OF SELECTED FRUITS

Fruit	Antioxidant Capacity
Strawberry	15.36
Plum	9.49
Orange	7.50
Grape, red	7.39
Kiwifruit	6.02
Grapefruit, pink	4.83
Grape, white	4.46
Banana	2.21
Apple	2.18

Fruit	Antioxidant Capacity
Tomato	1.89
Pear	1.34
Melon	0.97

Table adapted from Journal of Agricultural and Food Chemistry *44 (1996): 701–705.*

Dr. Zora Djuric's shortcut here is to eat the following:

- 2 vitamin C–rich fruits
- 2 other fruits

Serving size:
- medium-size piece of fruit, or
- 6 ounces 100 percent fruit juice, or
- ½ cup diced fruit, or
- ¼ cup dried fruit

In news reports, you'll often read about specific antioxidants. For years it was beta-carotene, but now lycopene is getting rave reviews. The unique table on pages 130–31, assembled by Catherine Rice-Evans in London, lists the antioxidant values of the very best antioxidants in the world and the foods in which you will find them.

ANTIOXIDANT POTENTIAL

The antioxidant power of each of the substances in the following table is compared to the antioxidant power of vitamin E. The actual technical name is "Trolox equivalent antioxidant activity." Trolox is a water-soluble vitamin E analog. So, as an example, quercetin would have 4.7 times the antioxidant capacity of vitamin E. That says quite a lot, since vitamin E is considered a powerful and effective antioxidant, especially in patients with heart disease.

FOODS WITH HIGHEST ANTIOXIDANT VALUES

Antioxidant	Antioxidant Value	Food
Quercetin	4.7	Onions, apple skin, berries, black grapes, tea, broccoli
Cyanidin	4.4	Grapes, raspberries, strawberries
Delphinidin	4.4	Eggplant skin
Epigallocatechin	3.8	Teas
Lycopene	2.9	Tomatoes
(Epi)catechin	2.4	Black grapes, red wine
P-coumaric acid	2.2	White grapes, tomatoes, spinach, cabbage, asparagus
Luteolin	2.1	Lemon, olive, celery, red pepper
Beta-cryptoxanthin	2.0	Mango, papaya, peaches, paprika, oranges
Beta-carotene	1.9	Carrots, sweet potato, tomatoes, paprika, green vegetables
Taxifolin	1.9	Citrus fruit

Step 7: Lower Oxidative Load

Antioxidant	Antioxidant Value	Food
Ferulic acid	1.9	Grains, tomatoes, spinach, cabbage, asparagus
Oenin	1.8	Black grapes, red wine
Lutein	1.5	Banana, satsuma peel, egg yolk, green vegetables
Apigenin	1.5	Celery, parsley
Zeaxanthin	1.4	Paprika, satsuma peel
Chrysin	1.4	Fruit skin
Alpha-carotene	1.3	Tomatoes, carrots, green vegetables
Kaempferol	1.3	Endive, leeks, broccoli, grapefruit, tea
Caffeic acid	1.3	White grapes, olives, spinach, cabbage, asparagus
Chlorogenic acid	1.3	Apples, pears, cherries, plums, tomatoes, peaches
Vitamin C	1.0	Fruits, vegetables
Vitamin E	1.0	Grains, nuts, oil
Echinenone	0.7	Artemia
Naringin	0.24	Citrus fruit peel
Astaxanthin	0.03	Salmon, food colorants, crab
Canthaxanthin	0.02	Carrots, kale, food colorants, red peppers

Adapted from Biochemical Society Transactions *24 (1996): 790–794.*

Supplement Warning

There is a great temptation to rely on vitamin supplements to make up for a poor diet. Nowhere will that gain you less than with breast cancer prevention. Studies show proof positive that real fruits and vegetables provide a powerful effect, whereas there's no such scientific proof that individual vitamins do the same. Singling out individual nutrients is called reductionism to the extreme. This strategy is also beginning to backfire. Research links beta-carotene supplements with increased risk of both lung and colon cancer. Some researchers believe that beta-carotene may block other important carotenes, of which there are nearly 500, from being absorbed, thus increasing the cancer risk by depriving the body of these important nutrients. Sloan-Kettering's breast cancer chief, Dr. Larry Norton, has shown that vitamin C can actually grow breast cancer cells in a petri dish. He recommends that his breast cancer patients take *no* vitamin supplements. Are there supplements you should consider? For protection against heart disease and neural tube defects, vitamins B6, B12, and folate are important and are often taken as supplements. Vitamin E helps to prevent fish oils from oxidizing in the body and protects against heart disease. However, there are no vitamin supplements known to protect against breast cancer. With the risk that some supplements, such as beta-carotene or vitamin C, could increase the cancer risk, the best advice is to get the maximum amount of vitamins from foods and then to supplement only after reviewing the need with your doctor.

HOW TO PREPARE VEGETABLES

Do you hate vegetables? Join the club. At last count perhaps 11 percent of Americans even ate the five daily servings of fruits and vegetables recommended. The lowest dietary compliance of all is for the consumption of fruits and vegetables: 140 million Americans are not eating the recommended amounts. Here's how we get around it at our house. We eat just a few really great-tasting vegetables like sweet potatoes that rank extremely high in antioxidants. We either sauté them or use a juicer (see below).

Mediterranean-Style

If you're really down on eating limp, mushy vegetables, here's a great no-compromise solution. This is the heart of the Mediterranean diet: vegetables sautéed in olive oil. This goes a long way toward satisfying your fat craving and can be a great deal healthier than a big dousing of low-fat but high-sugar salad dressings.

The Vita-Mixer

We use a Vita-Mixer to create a quick-to-eat, super powerful vegetable cocktail that will give you an instant buzz — guaranteed. The device is recommended by the Center for Science in the Public Interest in Washington, D.C. It crushes a plateful of vegetables and fruits so you can drink them in one simple serving. This is an easy task to perform when you come home in the evening. The Vita-Mixer has a 37,000 rpm, nearly two-horsepower, lawn mower–quality engine that can blast pulp, skins, even seeds into smithereens. Standard juicers leave juice so gritty you may find it unpleasant to drink. The Vita-Mixer produces a smooth puree. The manufacturer claims that all the nutrients are retained and that the machine liberates more of them than even our own digestive systems could. Our family mixes up several a day to get our entire antioxidant load in a quick, painless way. The device comes with a number of terrific recipes. Doctors at Strang suggest mixing one third of a head of broccoli and one quarter head of cabbage mixed with an equal amount of carrot juice.

Mongolian Barbecue

This is my favorite way to eat vegetables. Broccoli, cabbage, roots, onion, garlic, peppers . . . up to ten different vegetables are fried on a hot skillet . . . in water! Add teriyaki sauce and you'll find vegetables far crispier and tastier than you ever imagined. You'll truly love vegetables you always thought you hated!

Vegetable Danger

Many vegetarians believe that they eat a safer diet simply because they don't eat meat. Many replace meat in the diet with other foods rich in animal fat and cholesterol, such as cheese and whole dairy products. A recent study of nearly 11,000 health-conscious people, from meat eaters to vegetarians, showed that being a vegetarian didn't predict a decreased risk of disease, because many vegetarians still had diets high in calories and high in saturated fats. For instance, I'm always amused when I fly. I order a vegetarian meal. Pretty healthy, huh? The rice and beans look and taste terrific. They should, they are soaked in omega-6 fatty acids. I get an even bigger kick out of the Country Churn Whipped Butter. It even advertises "50% vegetable oil." However, the lead ingredient is a trans-fatty acid: partially hydrogenated soybean oil. Even more amusing is the All Natural Oatmeal Raisin Cookie, made from white flour, hydrogenated oils, and pure crystalline fructose, among the lead ingredients. You could eat a strictly vegetarian diet that is high in omega-6 fats, high in glucose load, and low in both omega-3 fats and soy. Many vegetarians do just that, but they will derive little preventive benefit.

Analysis

The simple truth is that most vegetables have a very non-specific role in fighting cancer. Vegetables do decrease the overall oxidative stress and do decrease the risk of breast cancer, but not in a dramatic way. If you have taken the measures already recommended in this book, then fruits and vegetables will add to the benefit. However, taken alone, without the other measures advocated in this book, they have only a modest effect because they do so little to interrupt the estrogen pathway. That's why results from a vegetarian diet have been disappointing. Too many vegetarians eat a diet loaded with ingredients that spike the estrogen pathway, from omega-6 fats and too little fiber to a high glucose load.

Recommendation

Eat five to nine fruits and vegetables per day that are near the high end of the tables provided in this chapter. Add a cup and a half of green tea per day. Green tea has one of the highest antioxidant values known and is now being used in clinical trials, including one at Memorial Sloan-Kettering.

STEP 8:

AVOID CHEMICAL

ESTROGENS

Imagine a super estrogen that is hundreds of times more powerful than the most potent natural estrogen. It fits precisely into the estrogen receptor, just like natural estrogens. Then imagine that it is included in many of the foods you eat, every day at every meal. This is the nightmare scenario of the chemical estrogen theory of breast cancer: chemicals in the environment that act just like an estrogen when they attach to the estrogen receptor on breast cells but provide a signal that is many times more powerful.

How could these chemicals still be in our food and water? The most pervasive chemical estrogen imitators are pesticides. DDT, although banned in 1974, has remained in the soil and water for nearly 25 years. Some pesticides may still be found in foods, since they are not routinely tested for, including those imported from other countries. Others make their way into the fat stores of animals and fish, where they are concentrated. The theory that chemicals in the environment may be a risk for breast cancer does have some support. A Mt. Sinai study of New York women showed that women with high levels of DDE (the breakdown product of DDT) had four times the risk of breast cancer than women with the lowest levels. In late 1997, P. V. M. Shekhar reported in the prestigious *Journal of the National Cancer Institute* that the pesticide DDT can "synergistically collaborate with estrogen." So while it need not have a powerful estrogenic effect on its own, combined with estrogen it can have a very potent effect.

The chemical estrogen theory is very alarming but has been very tough to prove. There is another camp with beliefs just as intense — that there is no connection at all, that these chemicals may even protect against breast cancer. It comes as little surprise that this latter camp is led by a major agricultural school. But they are joined by a prestigious group at Harvard. In fact the well-respected Harvard Nurses Health Study has failed to find any link between two of the most common organochlorines, DDT and PCBs, and breast cancer. The Harvard study has not made this a dead issue. The study simply tells us that blood levels don't correlate with cancer risk. However, fat, as we've seen, can concentrate these chemicals up to 700 times those found in the blood. With the debate at a seeming impasse, Dr. Barry Goldin of the Tufts University School of Medicine has taken chemical estrogens a quantum leap further. What Dr. Goldin showed is that by adding a combination of pesticides together, a more powerful mixture is created, far more powerful than any estrogen the body can make. Just look at three common pesticides: Endosulfan, which is mainly found in contaminated fruits and vegetables; and dieldrin and chlordane, which can be found in contaminated beef, lamb, chicken, freshwater fish, and some saltwater fish. The three together create what he calls "an alarming effect." Barry points out too that we're not exposed to just a single pesticide in the environment but to combinations just like these three. This helps greatly in solving the puzzle of how pesticides could lead to cancer. This concept is very similar to what researchers found after the Gulf War. No single agent caused Gulf War syndrome, but the combination of different toxic chemicals did. You'll recall that with Gulf War syndrome one panel of medical experts after another derided the idea of a common pattern to the illnesses being presented because combatants were not exposed to alarming levels of any one agent. So too with breast cancer: A mixture of pesticides creates a combination far more powerful than any estrogen. Still, this is a debate that remains very hot and is far from settled.

BREAST BENEFITS OF AVOIDING CHEMICAL ESTROGENS

The principal benefit of lowered chemical estrogen is that less energy is brought to the estrogen receptor. However, Marilie Gammon of Columbia University has shown that, under lab conditions, organochlorines can also increase estrogen production.

HOW TO CUT YOUR EXPOSURE
TO CHEMICAL ESTROGENS

Plant-Based Organic Diet

This is the safest and best way to reduce your exposure to chemical estrogens. If red meat has a high fat content, excess estrogen or chemical estrogens may be present in the fat. By eliminating meats, you cut a large source of animal fats that can store pesticides and other chemical estrogens. By eating organic foods from farms that have never used pesticides, you minimize the risk of ingesting chemical estrogens. The plants also provide protection against breast cancer with antioxidants and weak estrogens that block the estrogen receptor.

Lean Meats

There are meats that contain lesser amounts of injected or chemical estrogens. I look for organically produced beef and poultry. I trim poultry of skin and fat. By trimming these sources of fat before cooking, you ensure that you are not consuming potential carcinogens trapped in the fat. Also be sure to marinate your chicken before grilling, since unmarinated grilled chicken can still contain the same hefty share of the heterocyclic amines that red meats do. Look too for safer meats such as venison, turkey, quail, rabbit, and pheasant, all of which have far fewer chemical estrogens.

Lean Dairy

Dairy products carry organochlorines, largely in fat, so low-fat products are a much safer bet. Organically produced low-fat dairy products are the best of all. Organic soy milk is an even safer alternate.

Low-Risk Seafood

As great as omega-3 fatty acids are for breast protection, there is the added risk of chemical estrogens in the fat. Cold, deep saltwater fish, harvested as far away as possible from contaminated mainland estuaries, are safest. Those include tuna, sea bass, red snapper, arctic char, halibut, and orange roughy. Some of my favorites, unfortunately, are off the list. Those include the key fish off our summer home: bluefish, swordfish, lobster, and striped bass. Great Lakes fish and fish from inland waterways, and European rivers and inland waters, may also be risky. As a native of Boston and big fan of fish and fishing, I don't mean to be unduly alarming. The burden of proof, however, is on the seller. The fisheries industry says there is far less contamination now than in the past, but they need to provide the public with proof. Some innovative producers are making chemical-free fish. For instance a Norwegian fish farm has a deep, pollution-free fjord where it now produces salmon.

Organic Vegetables

Even in the United States, over a dozen pesticides can be sprayed on fruit or vegetables. My biggest concern is for pesticides, now outlawed in the United States, that may still be present on fruits and vegetables imported to America from foreign countries. You can remove many of the pesticides by a thorough washing, but organic products are unquestionably a safer bet.

Should you avoid fruits and vegetables if you can't get organic ones? A major review in the journal *Cancer* says the greater danger is avoiding fruits and vegetables altogether, because the gains so far outweigh the risks. The American Cancer Society point out that the consumption of five fruits and vegetables every day decreases the risk of breast cancer by 50 percent.

Block Chemical Estrogens

Since it's clearly impossible to avoid all chemical estrogens, and since every one of us still has chemical estrogens stored in our bodies, blocking their effect is the easiest strategy and may be the most effective. It's one you may have already elected to undertake to block the effect of natural estrogens. See the chapter "Step 1: Block the Estrogen Receptor" for information on how soy and flaxseed consumption can contribute to the estrogen-blocking effect.

So what should you do? Since the proof of this concept is far from convincing in the evidence presented to date, that leaves you, the consumer, with the possibility that the foods you eat are doing you real harm, but without the motivation to change foods or eating habits. How far should you go? With a young family, I would take the extra measure to limit chemicals in foods, especially given the dramatic rise in children's cancers and the large increased risk of breast cancer that is derived from childhood and adolescence. For a busy adult on the go, it's harder to make the case. Is it really worth all the effort? Will you really stick with the program? My advice is to take a few simple steps by being wise in your selection of meat, dairy, and fish products — and then to consider an estrogen receptor blocker.

There is an intensive effort under way to identify the most powerful chemical estrogens and to develop testing to find them in our food supply. The Environmental Protection Agency is pioneering the concept of the cumulative risk of multiple chemical estrogens; it is also developing tests for chemical estrogens in foods. Until those tests are regularly applied, the buyer must beware.

Recommendation

Until research is more conclusive, avoid meats, fish, and nonorganic produce that may be high in chemical estrogens, especially if you are a breast cancer survivor, are at high risk for breast cancer, or are an adolescent. For further information on reducing pesticide exposure, contact the Cornell Pesticide Management Education Program, an excellent resource with fact sheets and publications. They are located at 5123 Comstock Hall, Ithaca, NY 14583-0999 (phone: 607-255-1866).

STEP 9: DECREASE

BODY FAT

Excess body fat presents a risk of breast cancer throughout a woman's life, from childhood through menopause. Researchers at Memorial Sloan-Kettering are frankly surprised by the lack of attention paid to weight loss as a means of preventing cancer. Although there are many ways to weight control, there are several additional principles that are necessary to cut your cancer risk. Fortunately many of the measures you are already taking to control your weight, such as adding fiber, cutting your fat, and dropping your glucose load, will make a big impact on safe, effective fat loss. In fact you will find that fat loss is actually far easier using the measures recommended for control of cancer risk. You'll find weight loss a pleasure.

BREAST BENEFITS OF NORMAL BODY FAT

There are plenty of good reasons to be trim but a surprising number of reasons that being trim is good for your breasts. Abdominal fat is a veritable estrogen factory, so losing abdominal fat decreases estrogen production.

Girls with low body fat have later menarche. Women with low body fat slow the resumption of ovulation after breast-feeding and decrease the storage area for chemical estrogens. After menopause, a lower body fat decreases bad estrogen production and increases estrogen carrier production. For younger women, a lower body fat makes tumors far easier to find. Tumors are notoriously hard to find in young women with more than 15 to 20 percent excess body fat.

HOW TO DROP BODY FAT FOR MAXIMUM BREAST HEALTH

The most effective possible ways of controlling body fat are, not coincidentally, the most effective ways of decreasing the risk of breast cancer. The key is this: Let foods do the job for you. Why? Billions of people around the world perfectly control their weight simply by eating foods that keep them lean. Low-glucose, high-fiber foods are the heart of any such program. This is described in great detail in my last book, *Dr. Bob Arnot's Revolutionary Weight Control Program,* which outlines how foods act as drugs to help you lose weight. If you follow the full dietary program outlined in the following pages, you will be able to settle at the weight that gives you the least risk of breast cancer and the greatest degree of breast health. That program embodies the key principles of decreased glucose load, few saturated fats, and increased fiber.

Fiber is the foundation upon which any successful long-term weight-loss program is built. The University of Kentucky's Dr. James Anderson was one of the earliest to use gums and guars, agents that slow the digestion of food, with his patients. Even after 42 months of outpatient follow-up, Dr. Anderson's patients maintained an average 15-pound weight loss.

With its high fiber content, you'll find that soy adds to any weight-loss strategy. Soy protein also aids weight loss with its high fiber content, low glucose load, and the highest amount of the alertness-enhancing substance tyrosine of any food ever measured. Tyrosine plays a terrific role in maintaining your mental energy without the need for excess calories.

WHEN TO LOSE WEIGHT

The most dangerous time to gain weight is right at the menopause because fat serves as an enormous estrogen factory. So even though your ovaries stop producing estrogen, your fat stores produce huge amounts . . . enough so that many obese women feel few signs of the menopause. At the menopause is when you most want to control your weight. Earlier weight gain can also be quite harmful, especially in your twenties. Learning how to effectively control your weight in your late teens and early twenties is the best course of action. There are studies that show that premenopausal women who are frankly obese do have a lower risk of breast cancer — while they are premenopausal. That is because they have so much fat that it interferes with their menstrual cycles, thereby cutting estrogen production. However, their risk will soar once they pass menopause. Women who gain weight at the menopause run an even greater risk. They have none of the protection before menopause and all of the risk after menopause.

HOW MUCH SHOULD YOU WEIGH?

Since the real risk is upper body fat, the easiest way to determine whether you have too much fat is to measure a fold of skin next to your belly button. Much more than an inch and you're likely to have a body fat level high enough to raise your insulin level. This is a better target than shooting for a specific weight. Remember, you don't need to worry about being five to ten pounds over the ideal if you're eating great foods.

Recommendation

Try to get within 12 pounds of your ideal body weight. If you're doing everything else right, there's no need to be thinner.

STEP 10: LIMIT

ALCOHOL

Alcohol consumption is the most solidly established dietary factor related to cancer of the breast and one of the most powerful. The more you drink, the higher your risk. Little wonder! Alcohol is converted to acetaldehyde, which causes cancer in laboratory animals. Alcohol decreases the body's ability to use folic acid, which, in turn, adversely affects gene regulation. But most important, alcohol directly contributes to the estrogen effect. A National Cancer Institute study showed that alcohol elevates total estrogen levels and the amount of free estradiol that is available to attach to the breast. Abstinence decreases estrogen production. At the opposite extreme, large amounts of alcohol, especially when resulting in liver disease, greatly increase the risk of cancer. Here's why. The liver takes estrogen out of circulation. When the liver is damaged, estrogen levels may climb rapidly. One prime example is breast cancer in men, a cancer that is climbing rapidly in incidence. Most men who do not carry the cancer gene but are diagnosed with breast cancer have as their chief risk a high estrogen level resulting from alcohol damage to the liver. The large amounts of estrogen in their system are enough to cause the primitive breast structures in the male breast to grow. You can just imagine what it does to the female breast.

Dose

No alcohol is the safest dose. The specific effects of alcohol on pre- and postmenopausal women are described in the chapters "Breast Cancer Prevention Plan for Women with High Estrogen Levels" and ". . . for Women with Low Estrogen Levels." If you do drink, organic products, such as champagne, wine, beer, tequila, and vodka are clearly the safest, since they have the least risk of contamination or carcinogens.

Recommendation

If you're going to drink for your health, wait until you need it — that's well into your fifties — then drink sparingly.

STEP 11: INCREASE

VITAMIN D

Breast cancer rates vary directly with the amount of solar radiation. The colder, cloudier Northeast has a higher rate of breast cancer than the warmer, sunnier South. What's the connection? Exposure to sunlight helps the body manufacture vitamin D. Women in the Northeast manufacture less vitamin D because they are exposed to less natural sunlight, especially in the winter season. Here's how researchers made the connection. They graded a woman's exposure to the sun by the amount of skin damage she had suffered. Those with the most severe loss of elasticity in the skin had, paradoxically, the lowest risk of breast cancer! You might wonder why women didn't make up for the lack of vitamin D through sunlight by eating the right kinds of vitamin D–rich foods. A recent study from Massachusetts General Hospital showed that 59 percent of hospitalized patients had too little vitamin D in their bloodstream. That leads many experts to conclude that vitamin D deficiency is widespread in the general American population. The good news is that you can make a concerted effort to get the right amount of vitamin D from your diet and from proper exposure to sunlight.

BREAST BENEFITS OF VITAMIN D

Vitamin D is a potent inhibitor of a cell's ability to divide and grow. Vitamin D also helps breast cells to become more mature so they are less vulnerable to cancer-causing toxins.

Dose: A daily intake of 200 international units (IU) decreased risk of breast cancer by 36 percent. You may require even higher amounts of vitamin D to maintain strong bones. Here are the amounts recommended by the Institute of Medicine at the National Academy of Sciences:

Age	Recommended Amount of Vitamin D
19–50	200 IU
51–70	400 IU
71 plus	600 IU

As a result of a Massachusetts General Hospital study published in the March 19, 1998, *New England Journal of Medicine,* some experts believe that we should take even higher amounts of vitamin D, 800 to 1,000 IU. Why? Forty-six percent of those who ingested the daily recommended amount of vitamin D had too little vitamin D in their blood!

Sources: Most vitamin D should come from sunlight or real

food. There is no evidence that a vitamin D supplement has any effect on breast cancer rates.

Sunlight

Solar radiation can provide 75 percent of your daily vitamin D intake. You needn't stay out long, not enough to burn, and not when the sun is at its peak intensity, just enough for a healthy glow. Practically speaking, that means getting out for 15 minutes three times a week.

Food

Practically speaking, the easiest way to ingest vitamin D is in fortified breakfast cereals or milk. Eight ounces of milk has 100 IU. Each ounce of breakfast cereal has 50 IU.

Recommendation

Be sure to eat a minimum of 200 IU of vitamin D a day for breast cancer prevention . . . up to 1,000 IU to protect your bones. Get outdoors three times a week for at least 15 minutes, taking the usual precautions to avoid burning.

STEP 12:

EXERCISE

Exercise is such a powerful preventive factor that, were it a drug, it would be considered a major breakthrough. Women who have exercised their whole lives have altered their entire risk profile. Exercise intercepts the estrogen pathway at several critical junctures. Those women who are physically active when they are young adults are least likely to develop breast cancer, concludes Harvard's Rose Frisch. The most convincing study is that of more than 25,000 Norwegian women. The authors concluded that those who exercised at least four hours a week had a 37 percent lower risk of developing the disease. The more women exercised, the less likely they were to get breast cancer, the investigators found. The best results were found in those women who had already exercised three to five years. In America, a study at the University of Southern California of 1,000 women concluded that those who exercised 3.8 hours or more a week had less than half the breast cancer of those who remained inactive.

BREAST BENEFITS OF EXERCISE

There's little wonder that exercise is as effective as it is. Exercise blocks the estrogen effect by reducing estrogen production, delays the onset of menarche, prevents the accumulation of abdominal fat, reduces insulin levels, and raises the levels of good estrogen. The most exciting new development is that exercise may help to prevent recurrence of breast cancer. Weight gain seems to be a major predictor of recurrence, according to Pamela Goodwin of the University of Toronto.

Dose

In the Norwegian study previously noted, women exercised vigorously enough to raise their heart rates and break into a sweat and did so four or more hours a week. Contrast that to the recommendation by the Federal Centers for Disease Control of 20 minutes a day three times a week, which is not nearly enough. Many government and academic recommendations about exercise will tell you what they think you will do instead of what is the most beneficial. For heart health and breast health, four hours a week is the mark to shoot for. Clearly no one is going to hit that mark practicing an exercise they loathe unless they are extremely disciplined. Far better to aim for fun sports that you truly love, from tennis and mountain biking to roller blading and skiing. The easiest way to get those four hours is to find a great weekend activity that you can do for two or more hours each Saturday and Sunday. That leaves only two more hours during a busy week.

What about intensity? That's the big surprise. Clearly, high-intensity exercise helps to disrupt the estrogen pathway in young women in highly competitive sports. For middle-aged women, a moderate intensity of exercise helps to stabilize insulin levels and lower body fat better than more intense exercise.

Recommendation

Four or more vigorous hours of an aerobic activity you really love each week.

Part Three

BREAST CANCER
PREVENTION PLANS

ROAD MAP TO

BREAST CANCER

PREVENTION PLANS

The following chapters contain breast cancer prevention strategies. You'll find a full list of recommended steps in each of these chapters.

- Food plan for women with high estrogen levels.
- Food plan for women with low estrogen levels: This is for women who produce low amounts of estrogen, usually as a consequence of menopause.
- Breast cancer survivor diet: This is for women who have completed treatment for breast cancer.
- Supplements: This is a high-intensity chemoprevention program for high-risk women. Also, if you and your family can't commit to a full change in diet, you'll find a few simple daily supplements that should help you substantially cut the estrogen effect. Let me be clear about what I mean by supplements. Large doses of vitamins and of genistein are not recommended.

However, for three key ingredients of the breast cancer prevention diet, supplements are the most efficient way to ingest high doses. Those are fish oils, indole-3 carbinol, and estrogen blockers.

Should you choose to limit the number of steps you undertake to just the most effective, the steps advocated in these chapters are rated for their effectiveness, from one star (★) to five (★ ★ ★ ★ ★).

Following these chapters you'll find a chapter on dietary suggestions for girls and adolescents, a chapter on healthy cuisines, and a chapter of meal plans incorporating all of the recommendations of the breast cancer prevention diet.

BREAST CANCER PREVENTION PLAN FOR WOMEN WITH HIGH ESTROGEN LEVELS

(Before Menopause)

The premenopausal years are when most women palpably feel the risk of breast cancer for the first time. They see friends or mothers die of the disease. It is a frightening time, and that fear usually turns to action — if there is any action to take. If you are a younger woman there is a great deal that you can do to avoid breast cancer. For most of you, it is not likely that you will see the results pay off until the postmenopausal years, when the greatest number of breast cancer cases develop.

★ ★ ★ ★ ★ DRINK SPARINGLY

Alcohol has its strongest effect on a premenopausal female. Each daily drink increases the risk of breast cancer by 11 percent. Alcohol works by increasing estrogen levels in the blood. Clearly, in the premenopausal years, when the body produces large amounts of estrogen, alcohol can have a very large effect. The greatest effect is for women who begin drinking before thirty. Women under thirty run the biggest risks and derive the least benefit from alcohol. Alcohol in younger women also increases the risk of depression, suicide, poisoning, cirrhosis of the liver, and accidental death. This is also when the risk of coronary artery disease is extremely low and there is little rationale for drinking to prevent heart disease.

★★★★★ BLOCK ESTROGEN

Estrogen blockers play their most positive preventive role in premenopausal women. While there are many questions about soy usage in adolescents and postmenopausal women, a healthy daily dose of soy is what appears to keep hundreds of millions of women in the Far East free from cancer. After evaluating all the risks and benefits of soy as detailed in the chapter "Step 1: Block the Estrogen Receptor," consider eating 35 to 60 grams of soy a day, or 25 grams of flax, if you have never had breast cancer. Since soy is one of the highest-quality proteins in nature, you may simply want to substitute soy for most of your other protein. Using soy during pregnancy or while nursing is covered in the chapter "Daughters." Since both breast-feeding and pregnancy provide on their own protection against breast cancer, consuming soy is not as critical during those times. Three studies have shown a reduced risk for premenopausal breast cancer with soy consumption. If you are at extremely high risk of breast cancer and carry the BRCA1 or BRCA2 gene, you should determine if an estrogen-blocking drug is appropriate by consulting with top experts at a National

Cancer Institute–designated comprehensive cancer center. Raloxifene is not approved for use by premenopausal women. Tamoxifen has been reviewed by the FDA for use by premenopausal women and has a low side-effect profile for women under 50.

★ ★ ★ ★ ★ EXERCISE

This is one of the few absolutely proven steps to prevent breast cancer. Intense exercise cuts estrogen production and may interfere with menstrual cycles. This substantially cuts the estrogen effect. However, adolescent girls should not overdo it, since exercise physiologists are concerned that extremely vigorous exercise can stop menstrual periods altogether, possibly leading to extensive bone loss.

★ ★ ★ ★ AVOID OMEGA-6 FATS

A lifelong habit of avoiding omega-6 fats will protect your breasts from the powerful booster effect these fats inflict.

★ ★ ★ ★ EAT FISH OR TAKE FISH OIL

Fish in the diet is a good long-term preventive strategy, provided the fish are low in chemical estrogens. If you won't eat fish or are at a high risk of breast cancer, then supplementing your diet with 10 grams of fish oil a day is worth discussing with your doctor. As a young woman, if you avoid omega-6 fats, you have less need for fish oil capsules, since you may not need to compensate with large amounts of omega-3 fats.

★ ★ ★ ★   CONTROL BODY FAT

Weight gained from the age of 18 on creates a striking risk for breast cancer. In fact many of the other risk factors such as a high-fat, high-calorie diet or lack of exercise may all exert their risk primarily through building excess body fat. The increased risk of excess body fat will not be apparent until after you reach menopause. However, it's not worth waiting until menopause to lose the weight. The most powerful studies show that it's weight gained early in adulthood that does the greatest damage.

★ ★ ★   DROP GLUCOSE LOAD

A high insulin level is a risk even for thin premenopausal women. Since a high glucose load is likely to lead to the kind of apple-shaped obesity where fat is stored around the abdomen, instead of the buttocks and thighs, and lifelong weight problems, a diet low in glucose load makes sense.

★ ★ ★   ADD FIBER

Since the premenopausal years are when your body produces the largest amounts of estrogen, trapping that estrogen with fiber is an important step. Thirty-five grams of fiber is the minimum. If you can work your way up to 50 grams you will achieve a spectacular ability to control your hunger and your weight.

★★★ DROP YOUR OXIDANT LOAD

This drops your overall risks of initiating cancer as well as helping with lifelong weight control. Nine-a-day fruits and vegetables gives you your maximum advantage.

★★ EAT CRUCIFEROUS VEGETABLES

With large circulating levels of estrogen, it's important to channel as much into good estrogen as possible. Cruciferous vegetables do just that. For women at high risk, supplementing with indole-3 carbinol supplements produces a pronounced effect. The starting dose is 300 milligrams a day.

★ AVOID CHEMICAL ESTROGENS

The younger you are, the less likely it is that you have been exposed to major amounts of chemical estrogens, but the more vigilant you should be about avoiding future exposure. Until more is known, avoiding foods likely to contain pesticide residue and other chemical estrogens is a wise move.

A note about pregnancy: New research shows that low amounts of estrogen during pregnancy may lead to miscarriage. For that reason you may not want to cut the estrogen effect while you are pregnant. This is an important point to cover with your obstetrician.

BREAST CANCER PREVENTION
PLAN FOR WOMEN WITH
LOW ESTROGEN LEVELS

(After Menopause)

The majority of breast cancer is diagnosed in postmenopausal women. Many of the preventive steps you take as a younger woman will pay off here. If you have not taken any of those steps as a young woman, you will want to begin a more rigorous prevention program. Although ovarian estrogen production drops dramatically after menopause, estrogen produced by the adrenal glands and in body fat and muscle can still supply a significant amount, especially in Western women. One study found that British postmenopausal women had estrogen levels 171 percent higher than those of Chinese women.

★★★★★ CONTROL BODY FAT

Since body fat is the key source of estrogen production for postmenopausal women, this is the most important and dangerous source of estrogen. This evidence comes from 121,000 women enrolled in the Harvard Nurses Health Study. Overweight postmenopausal women had 50 to 100 percent more estrogen than lean women. Weight gain at menopause and after appears to cause the greatest risk because it is the largest contributor to estrogen production. Obesity is also associated with a larger tumor size at the time of diagnosis, more spread to lymph nodes, and poorer survival. Both a low glucose load and exercise help to control your weight and your breast cancer risk.

★ ★ ★ ★ ★ EXERCISE

After the menopause, moderate exercise may be the most helpful. Walking at a modest speed of 18 to 20 minutes a mile burns fat and increases the body's sensitivity to insulin, so that less is required, according to a study by Katarina Borer of the University of Michigan. This also helps to burn off extra body fat.

★ ★ ★ ★ EAT FISH OR TAKE FISH OIL

This will rapidly increase your ratio of omega-3 to omega-6 fats. Since it takes about three years for your body to rid itself of omega-6, you may want to protect yourself by taking a higher dose of fish oils for those three years. That's why you may want to consider the full 10-grams-per-day dose of fish oils while you wash omega-6 fats out of your system. What I mean by "washing out" is that over the course of three years on a diet very low in omega-6 fats, those omega-6 fats will be used up by the body and gradually replaced by healthier fats.

★★★ BLOCK ESTROGENS

Some postmenopausal women still make large amounts of estrogen. Those are women with a high amount of body fat or a high-calorie, high-fat, lower-fiber diet. Other women are taking estrogen as part of hormone replacement therapy (HRT) and drink alcohol on a daily basis. Still others have large amounts of chemical estrogen concentrated in their breast fat. If you are counted among them, you may still benefit from an estrogen receptor blocker's ability to displace these estrogens from estrogen receptors. Because of the possibility that soy may stimulate the breast, you want to be certain to be within the "estrogen window." That is, paradoxically, very low doses of soy are as likely to stimulate the breast as are huge amounts. To remain within this window of soy consumption, aim for between 35 and 60 grams of soy per day. Soy is also considered a substitute for HRT in that it has a protective effect on bone and heart and diminishes the symptoms of menopause. The other alternative is the drug raloxifene. It is FDA approved for postmenopausal women to prevent osteoporosis. If you're not going to take HRT, this is a great alternative because it helps to preserve bone, lowers your cholesterol level, and may cut your risk of breast cancer as much as 90 percent after just 30 months of use. Tamoxifen has a higher side-effect and risk profile than raloxifene but could be considered by women at very high risk. Adding aromatase inhibitors may reduce the risk of breast cancer an *additional* 90 percent. For high-risk postmenopausal women, the combination of an aromatase inhibitor and raloxifene may be extremely promising — this combination could reduce the risk of breast cancer by 99 percent, bringing the risk level close to the low one that males currently have.

★★★ DRINK SPARINGLY

Alcohol has less of an effect on postmenopausal females, because there is less estrogen to boost. So in the years when heart disease is looming as a far greater risk, you may want to consider a glass of red wine.

In middle-aged and older women, several drinks a week gives you significant protection against heart disease with only a minimal increased risk of breast cancer, but only for women who are already at risk for heart disease. The table below gives a closer look at the actual risks for women in this age group as presented in a recent *New England Journal of Medicine* article.

ALCOHOL AND HEALTH RISK (BY PERCENTAGE)

Condition	No drinks	Less than a drink per day	1 drink per day	2–3 drinks per day
Cirrhosis	4	4.3	7.7	10.4
Breast cancer	30	33	37	45
Heart disease, no known risk	78	62	59	67
Heart disease, known risk	276	200	156	170

As you can see, at less than a drink per day there is only a marginal increase in breast cancer risk with a substantial drop in deaths from heart disease. If you are at risk for heart disease, there is an even larger drop in death with a single drink a day, with a small increased risk in breast cancer. With two to three drinks, some of the heart protective effects begin to fade and the breast cancer rate climbs even higher, as does that for cirrhosis.

However, the rules change if you are taking hormone replacement therapy because alcohol boosts the estrogen levels in the bloodstream, which increases the risk of breast cancer.

With HRT, drinking alcohol can triple the amount of circulating estrogens. Elizabeth S. Ginsburg, M.D., from the department of obstetrics and gynecology, Brigham and Women's Hospital, Boston, conducted a double-blind, crossover study of 24 postmenopausal women to determine the effects of moderate alcohol consumption on the circulating level of estradiol. The study reported that estradiol levels increased by 327 percent following alcohol ingestion in women on estrogen replacement therapy. What's more, significant increases in estradiol were detected within 10 minutes after drinking, when blood alcohol levels were still low. The great fear is that HRT plus alcohol use increases the risk of breast cancer to greater than that of either alone. What's even worse is that the effects of alcohol accumulate: The more you drink in a given period, the higher the estradiol level. There are some who believe much of the risk of HRT lies in its combination with alcohol.

If you do consider HRT, consider a very low dose. A new study in the *Archives of Internal Medicine* shows that women get the bone-sparing and heart-protective effects of estrogen with fewer side effects even if they take half the usual dose — 0.3 milligrams instead of the usual 0.625 milligrams.

One easy way to have it all may be to skip your estrogen therapy on the days you drink so that there is no boost in your blood level. That way you're getting the heart protection of estrogens one day and of alcohol the others. You'll want to discuss this with your doctor.

If you're considering HRT as short-term treatment of menopausal symptoms and are concerned about breast cancer, be reassured that the actual risk isn't apparent until 10 years of therapy have been completed . . . especially if you don't drink and aren't at high risk for breast cancer. However, as more and more medications that protect the heart, bones, *and* breast come on the market, I believe you'll ultimately elect to replace HRT with one of them for longer-term preventive therapy. That means you can start taking HRT now for symptomatic relief, with a view to switching to the selective estrogen receptor modulator (SERM) of your choice as they come on the market. SERMs are designed to have all the good effects of estrogen with none of the bad. Raloxifene is a successful early example.

★ ★ ★ EAT CRUCIFEROUS VEGETABLES

With the far lower production of estrogen, there's less "bad" estrogen that cruciferous vegetables can influence. They're still helpful and contain lots of antioxidants to lower oxidant load.

★★★ DROP GLUCOSE LOAD

A low glucose load will go a long way toward protecting you against the weight gain that often occurs with menopause.

★★★ DROP OXIDANT LOAD

A high fruit and vegetable diet still remains the best way to block the initiation of cancer.

★★★ AVOID OMEGA-6 FATS

Even though overall estrogen production has decreased, there can still be a substantial booster effect from eating bad fats. You may substitute olive oils or fish oil. If your whole life you have eaten a diet high in omega-6 fats, now you can lower your risk more quickly by taking fish oils on a daily basis.

★★ ADD FIBER

Fiber's primary importance after the menopause is to control weight and protect against heart disease. Since there is far less estrogen produced, there is less importance given to "trapping" estrogen with fiber.

★ AVOID CHEMICAL ESTROGENS

Most of your exposure to chemical estrogens will come from what you ate when pesticides were in heavy use, prior to the early 1970s. Since those levels can be pretty high, protecting yourself against chemicals already in your body is key. Both estrogen blockers and a diet rich in omega-3 fats will help you blunt the effect of chemical estrogens.

BREAST CANCER PREVENTION
PLAN FOR BREAST
CANCER SURVIVORS

Breast cancer survivors are routinely being put on diets to prevent recurrence. These diets are radically different in purpose from the general breast cancer prevention diet. Because stray cancer cells may still be present, the diet's job is actually to help fight and destroy cancer cells and to prevent regrowth over a very short time frame — as little as several months. Diet is clearly not a substitute for chemotherapy, radiation, or surgery, but it is being used at top centers to supplement them. As I've mentioned, flax is being given to cancer patients even before surgery to shrink tumor size. Since treatment programs are individualized, you will want to go over your nutritional treatment with your oncologist or an oncologist who deals with nutrition at a top cancer center.

BREAST BENEFITS OF DIET

Beyond the basic benefits of cutting the estrogen effect, researchers hope for even more aggressive cancer-fighting properties from diet, including the following: decrease tumor size, wall off tumor growth, cut off the fuel for further growth, shut down further genetic damage.

The recommendations here are divided into two parts. First, those for which there are no reservations because they are universally accepted to be safe and effective. Second, because this crosses over from pure prevention into part of an intensive medical plan, those recommendations that you will want to discuss with your doctor to be certain they are part of a solid overall treatment plan.

Recommended without hesitation:

★ ★ ★ ★ ★ DON'T DRINK

Alcohol is such a clear and well-established risk that it makes sense to drink sparingly or not at all.

★ ★ ★ ★ ★ AVOID OMEGA-6 FATS

Cutting the booster effect to a bare minimum by avoiding polyunsaturated fats is crucial. Substituting omega-3 fats may have a strong synergistic effect.

★ ★ ★ ★ ★ EXERCISE

Exercise plays a big part in improving your sense of well-being after surviving cancer. It will also help you drop your estrogen production.

★ ★ ★ ★ ★ TAKE FISH OIL

Changes are early and dramatic with fish oil. This is an aggressive measure that quickly changes the biology of your breast. Many cancer centers now firmly recommend this. The only question is dose, since high doses have been linked to bleeding. Ten milligrams is a safe dose in terms of bleeding. Sloan-Kettering and UCLA both include fish oils as part of regular and experimental protocols.

★ ★ ★ ★ CONTROL BODY FAT

This has the added benefit of making recurrences easier to detect early.

★ ★ ★ ★ AVOID HRT

Avoiding HRT makes sense because you cut the estrogen load on your system. If you really want to take an estrogen for menopausal symptoms, then consider raloxifene or soy.

★ ★ ★ ★ ADD FIBER

Trapping estrogen in the bowel and preventing recirculation makes the most sense if you are still exposed to near normal levels of estrogen. The fiber will also help with weight control.

★ ★ ★ ★ ★ BLOCK ESTROGEN RECEPTORS

Estrogen-blocking drugs are the most effective means of cutting the estrogen effect.

Tamoxifen is the most frequently prescribed estrogen blocker. Five-year survival figures are close to 90 percent when given with chemotherapy for breast cancer survivors.

Raloxifene poses an interesting alternative. It appears to protect against breast cancer, with a 77 percent decrease in cancer after just 18 months' use in women who did not have cancer when they began the trial, and as much as 90 percent after 30 months. Doctors are awaiting clinical trials to determine what use it may have in breast cancer and whether it poses any risk to the ovaries.

Soy: This is the area of greatest nutritional contention in women who have survived breast cancer. The question remains whether soy is a suitable estrogen receptor blocker once a patient has stopped taking tamoxifen or completed treatment. Since there are no suitable clinical trials to answer the question, it remains unanswered.

Since soy can act as a weak estrogen, many oncologists are squeamish about prescribing it for women who have low estrogen states as a result of breast cancer therapy or menopause. *Any* estrogenic effect could be potentially harmful, and the weak estrogenic effect of soy is included. Many doctors think it's playing with fire. Genistein, the most active component, can act as both an estrogen and an anti-estrogen. It's difficult to predict how it will act and it can act in both ways at the same time in one person.

A look to Asian women, however, shows no sign of a problem has ever been detected in breast cancer survivors. Soy has other anticancer properties, such as its effects as an antioxidant and its ability to block new blood vessel growth.

Clearly, premenopausal women with fully functioning ovaries and high levels of estrogen production might benefit. For postmenopausal patients, few doctors dare make any kind of prescriptive advice. For that reason you will want to review this with your oncologist.

If you go the soy route, remember that the risk, if any, is in eating too little soy. For that reason, you'll want to make the full commitment to 35 or 60 grams a day.

Receptor status: Breast cancer cells may also have estrogen receptors — breast cancer cells that have estrogen receptors are called estrogen receptor positive or ER positive. That means that estrogen can spur further growth of the tumor by attaching to the receptor so that estrogen blockers may be an effective adjunct to treatment.

Flaxseed: Since proof of flaxseed as an estrogen blocker is just now being published, you will need to review taking it with your doctor.

★★★ DROP GLUCOSE LOAD

The cross talk between insulin and estrogen receptors is pure bad news, since together they create an even stronger estrogen effect. Using a lowered glucose load to lower insulin decreases the synergy between estrogen and insulin to lower the estrogen effect.

★★★ EAT CRUCIFEROUS VEGETABLES

Since "bad" estrogens may actually induce cancers by attaching to a cell's DNA, cruciferous vegetables are an important part of the plan.

★★★ LOWER CALORIES

Sloan-Kettering recommends a low-calorie diet. This may seem counterintuitive for cancer survivors trying to nourish themselves, but Dr. Moishe Shike strongly believes that excess calories may be potent cancer promoters in these women. He has no reservations about this diet in early-stage cancers. By low-calorie, Dr. Shike means about 1,500 calories — not an overly restrictive calorie intake. Rita Mitchell, the nutritionist who prepared the meal plans listed in this book, feels this may be too low for some women to feel good and remain active. Your nutritionist can help determine what the right number of calories is for your diet.

★★★ DROP OXIDANT LOAD

Since this is the only available measure to stop the constant toxic barrage on your DNA, a nine-a-day fruit and vegetable diet, emphasizing those highest in antioxidants, is critical.

★★★ AVOID CHEMICAL ESTROGENS

Surgeons at Sloan-Kettering strongly advise their patients to avoid eating risky fish and meats that may contain chemical estrogens. For a breast cancer survivor, avoiding these chemicals is vitally important until more is known about their risks.

Recommended in consultation with your oncologist
or as part of a trial:

★★★ TAKE INDOLE-3 CARBINOL
SUPPLEMENTS

Since "bad" estrogens may play a role in both cancer initiation and growth, a full dose of I3C capsules should be considered. Since dosing is still being worked out, this is considered experimental. However, you will want to take a minimum of 300 milligrams a day, the lowest dose considered effective. In some trials 500 milligrams is now being used as a daily dose.

Gene status: For those women who carry BRCA1, BRCA2, and other yet to be discovered genetic mutations, most serious researchers do not believe that diet can prevent cancers from growing. Far more powerful genetically engineered tools are likely to be necessary, combined with a powerful estrogen receptor drug, either tamoxifen or raloxifene. Presently, for women at very high risk of breast cancer, there is much more hard clinical data on tamoxifen than there is on raloxifene.

Recommendation

My recommendation is to participate in an established clinical protocol so that you can receive all the advantages of careful observation and the encouragement to observe the diet strictly.

INTENSIVE INTERVENTION

SUPPLEMENTS

Many lead researchers are concentrating the most powerful components of foods into high-powered supplements in an effort to prevent breast cancer. For those at highest risk, this program combines the most powerful anticancer supplements on the market. This is an incredibly simple program requiring only a few minutes of your day.

PREMENOPAUSAL

★★★★ Fish oil capsules: 10 grams a day
★★★★ Estrogen blockers

Soy protein powder: 60 grams a day
or
Flax: 25 grams a day
or

Consider an estrogen-blocking drug (tamoxifen or raloxifene) as part of an established clinical trial if you are at very high risk.

★★★★ No alcohol
★★★★ Exercise
  ★★★ Indole-3 carbinol: 500 milligrams a day
  ★★★ No omega-6 fats

POSTMENOPAUSAL

Since the estrogen pathway has diminished substantially in its intensity by the end of menopause, a supplemented strategy is less important than a strong, balanced diet. There is also concern about soy supplements in women with low estrogen production, so these are not included.

★★★★ No omega-6 fats
★★★★ Fish oil capsules: 10 grams a day
★★★★ Indole-3 carbinol: 500 milligrams a day

Estrogen-Blocking Drug

If you wish to avoid HRT and also decrease your risk of osteoporosis, consider raloxifene, an estrogen blocker that decreases your risk of breast cancer and helps protect bone.

Researchers recommend a supplement strategy as part of an established clinical trial. I believe they are right and so recommend a supplement strategy for women at high risk as part of a clinical trial.

The supplement strategy may ultimately be what most American women choose. Here's why. Many doctors don't believe that most Americans will adapt to a largely plant-based, high-fiber, low-glucose-load diet. The evidence is on their side. Vanishingly few Americans are willing to eat fruits and vegetables, and even fewer are likely to eat a truly vegetarian diet. For that reason, a unique new strategy is emerging in cancer centers across the country that involves using powerful supplements and a few food changes to bring about a dramatic drop in the estrogen effect and its booster effect. Since dietary habits are so difficult to change, why not just offer a few food substitutions? That's exactly the approach that several top centers are taking. The bottom line is that you have to be able to eat a simple diet, year in and year out. I would far rather see you embrace the foods described in the previous chapters, but if you can't, consider this program.

DETERMINING YOUR LEVEL OF RISK

Read through the following descriptions of risk to determine your own level of risk.

Average

You are at average risk if you have no family history of breast cancer or if just one first- or second-degree relative contracted breast cancer after age 50. (First-degree relatives are sisters, daughters, and mothers. Second-degree relatives are first cousins, grandmothers, and aunts.)

Moderately Increased

You are at moderately increased risk if you have at least one first- or second-degree relative who was diagnosed with breast cancer before age 50 or if two relatives on the *same* side of the family were diagnosed with breast cancer.

High

You have a high degree of risk if three or more first- or second-degree relatives on the same side of the family were diagnosed with breast cancer or ovarian cancer.

Extremely High

You carry the BRCA gene mutation or already have contracted breast cancer. A woman with an inherited copy of either BRCA1 or BRCA2 has an 87 percent risk of developing breast cancer by age 70, with a much greater risk in the pre-menopausal years.

DAUGHTERS:

Intergenerational

Breast Cancer

Prevention

The strongest effects of diet on breast cancer may be the earliest. The development of the human breast begins during the first few months in the uterus. The hormones and toxins it is exposed to then and for the next two decades will have an enormous impact on the development of breast cancer. The frightening proposition is that this could be a cancer developed in childhood and adolescence that shows up in middle age.

The failure of many breast cancer prevention trials in American women has prompted doctors at Harvard and other institutions to study intergenerational breast cancer prevention. This is the hottest field in breast cancer prevention today. It is called intergenerational because women aim their preventive efforts at their daughters and granddaughters as well as themselves. In this chapter we'll look at what you could do, what you should do, and where the risks outweigh the advantages. Clearly, any lifelong measure requires the most meticulous care imaginable. With fast-developing tissues, the wrong move could be bad news.

Why do scientists believe that early development is so important? Here are the clues. After the atom bombs were dropped on Hiroshima and Nagasaki, breast cancers developed far more frequently among young women who were in their teens and early twenties when the bombs fell. Adult survivors did not show excess breast cancer development. The assumption is that the immature breast tissue of these young women was far more vulnerable than that of older women. What evidence is there that early diet has an effect? Although women who come to the United States from countries with lower risks of breast cancer, such as Japan, do develop a higher rate of breast cancer here, they don't reach the same high rate as American women. It is their daughters and granddaughters who do reach the same high rate as other American women. The smart money says that the foods these second- and third-generation Japanese-American women ate in America from early childhood accounted for the increased risk. Most serious researchers believe that prevention of breast cancer should begin very early. So do breast cancer survivors.

Deborah McCurdy, the breast cancer survivor we met earlier in this book, has her entire family on the breast cancer diet. "My whole family eats this way now — I've got four kids, 14, 10, 8, and 5, and they know all about fats, the right kinds of fats, the wrong kinds of fats, and it's just not a big deal. It's good to start in childhood. Diet may be critical in childhood and adolescence in taking steps to prevent cancer and other diseases. They start eating right early and they just follow it through as they get older. My big concern is that I just don't want my children to go through what I went through. And I want to be around to see them grow up and be healthy. This diet is a good way to do that."

ROAD MAP

We'll look at each stage of development and at the most interesting and important interventional strategies. When do you start? Does a mother have to drink soy milk while she is pregnant and nursing? Do young girls have to restrict their intake of fat? Do adolescents need to eat a vegetarian diet to prevent cancer? You can't start too early — or can you? Here's a look at the measures you can take for yourself and for your daughter or granddaughter.

THE FETUS

The excess estrogen that a fetus is exposed to in utero does increase the child's risk of breast cancer. Twins, who are exposed to higher than normal amounts of estrogen during pregnancy, have higher rates of breast cancer later in life, concludes Nancy Potischman of the National Cancer Institute. Women who have eclampsia or preeclampsia, conditions with low estrogen levels, give birth to babies who were exposed to much less estrogen in utero. These children have 50 percent to 80 percent less breast cancer risk than infants born of normal pregnancies. Since these conditions are dangerous to mother and child, you wouldn't want to mimic that condition. How else could you block estrogen? With estrogen blockers such as soy. In fact, the most interesting and alluring food to eat during pregnancy is soy because of the possibility that the estrogen effect could be cut even before the baby was born. In laboratory animals the idea works. Genistein fed to pregnant rats yielded a whopping 50 percent reduction in breast cancer in the offspring. "The results should be the same in humans because rat and human mammary glands are very similar," says Coral Lamartiniere of the University of Alabama at Birmingham.

Dr. Ken Setchell has already begun looking at this phenomenon in humans. He wanted to see if soy that mothers ate had any way of getting to the fetus. He compared samples of blood from the mother and from the fetus. Preliminary results show that the active ingredient, genistein, does cross the placenta, and levels can be measured in amniotic fluid. That means it gets to the fetus after the mother has consumed it. Is that something American mothers should try? The only absolute proof would come from long-term, placebo-controlled studies, but those would be way too costly and time-consuming to conduct. That leaves us only with the experience of Asian women who eat soy before, during, and after their pregnancies. Neither they nor their offspring seem to suffer any bad effects. The theoretical warning is for pregnant women because of the fear of retarding the growth of the fetus. In practice, this has never been observed in humans. If you're pregnant and thinking about taking soy for its estrogen effect, you'll want to discuss this carefully with your obstetrician. No supplements recommended in this book should be taken during pregnancy until thoroughly discussed with your obstetrician.

Recommendation

Monitor future research carefully.

INFANTS

There are two key preventive strategies to consider: breast-feeding and soy formula. The longer a child is breast-fed, the lower her chance of developing breast cancer; at the same time the mother lowers her own risk. Breast-fed infants have a 15 to 30 percent lower chance of developing breast cancer both before and after menopause. Breast-feeding also unloads from the breast chemical estrogens into breast milk. This is a risk-free and smart strategy to get your daughter off on the right foot and to drop your own risk of breast cancer. Breast-feeding also completes the maturation of the mother's breast so that it becomes less vulnerable to radiation, secondhand smoke, and other environmental hazards as well as estrogen. The American Academy of Pediatrics now strongly recommends breast-feeding for a full twelve months, with infants taking no other drink or solids for the first six months. This protects babies from a variety of ailments and protects their mothers against premenopausal breast cancer and ovarian cancer. American women who breast-feed for a total of two years decrease their risk 20 to 30 percent.

Infants drinking a soy formula have circulating blood levels of weak estrogens that are 13,000 to 20,000 times higher than their own estrogen production. This makes the use of these formulas controversial. They are having a biological effect, but is it strongly protective or harmful? That amount is six to eleven times more than is required to lengthen the menstrual cycle in premenopausal women — in other words a very powerful dose. In rats, this has proved very helpful. "We've been able to show that injections of genistein given to rats during either the neonatal or prepubertal periods results in about a 50 percent decrease of mammary tumors in adults," says Coral Lamartiniere. Soy formulas have been used now for 30 years without reports of adverse circumstances. Of U.S. babies, 29 percent consume soy formulas. Growth charts do not show growth retardation from soy, nor is bone development different. However, recent concern about potential adverse consequences has caused enough alarm in the United Kingdom and Australia for soy formula consumption to drop by half.

Recommendation

Consider breast-feeding to decrease your risk and that of your child. Consider soy only after careful discussion with your pediatrician.

CHILDHOOD TO MENARCHE

Milk duct cells are the most unusual in the body because they are the only human cells that are not fully differentiated at birth. Because they are in this immature state, they are more easily stimulated by estrogen to divide and more susceptible to harm from cancer-causing substances. Only after a full-term pregnancy do these cells become fully mature. That leaves them at risk for at least the first two decades of a woman's life. When a woman is an adolescent or in her twenties, the milk duct breast cells are especially vulnerable to these changes. If a lifetime of estrogen exposure increases the risk of breast cancer, then those girls reaching menarche earliest would have the highest risk. In fact that proves to be correct: Those girls who begin menstruation at 14 or before have a 30 percent increased chance of breast cancer. Early menarche is bad news right across the board. Girls with early menarche, before 12 years of age, have significantly higher serum estradiol and lower sex hormone binding globulin concentrations, and those differences remain an astounding 20 to 30 years later. This induces a higher degree of breast duct proliferation. That's why more and more researchers are looking for an early start at preventing breast cancer, to prevent risk that can last a lifetime. Girls with early menarche not only start producing estrogen earlier, they produce more estrogen. Why? The earlier menarche comes, the more likely that full and regular menstrual cycles begin early too. With later menarche the opposite is true. Periods are often irregular for several years more, which means that full estrogen production is delayed well past menarche. A Finnish study proved just that point. Girls with menarche earlier than age 12 had ovulatory cycles 80 percent of the time within one to two years. By contrast, in girls with menarche at age 13 or later, it was about four and a half years before even 50 percent of their cycles were ovulatory. So, as you can see, early menarche has long-term effects on lifelong estrogen production. Can food make a difference?

Harvard's Dr. Graham Colditz is quoted as saying: "Simple dietary modification may contribute to delay in menarche and substantial reduction in lifetime risk of breast cancer." Childhood is an excellent time to establish a really healthful diet. Learning to eat a healthy diet as a child makes the job infinitely easier as an adult. Ernst Wynder, president of the American Health Foundation, says that basic tastes are acquired by age six.

Avoid Omega-6 Fats

Courtney and I try to avoid feeding our own children polyunsaturated fats of any kind. This prevents the breast cells from ever acquiring the fats that cause the estrogen booster effect.

Lower Glucose Load

We also try to keep all our carbohydrates in the low glycemic range. The syndrome of upper body obesity and high insulin levels is linked to a high risk of breast cancer. A group of French researchers proposes lowering glucose load in teenagers to prevent the syndrome before it starts. This also helps enormously in keeping weight under control, as will a high-fiber diet.

Eat Enough Fiber

Fiber is the best single guard against bingeing in adolescence. Girls who eat too little fiber have an earlier menarche.

Lower-Calorie Diet

The Norwegian study cited, of women born between 1930 and 1932 and exposed to famine at about the age of menarche, reflected a 13 percent decrease in death from breast cancer. This protection works all the way through the adult years, well past menopause. Clearly this "experiment" was unintentional and excessive, but a moderate number of calories go a long way toward controlling weight and estrogen production. This is made far easier by a low-glucose-load diet that is high in fiber.

Less Body Fat

Girls with excess body fat reach menarche earlier than thinner girls. Overweight kids become overweight adults, who then produce large amounts of estrogen throughout their adult lives.

More Physical Activity

Preadolescent girls who engage in strenuous activity such as running, swimming, and ballet have later menarche than girls who do not. Girls who exercise also produce less estrogen, have a lower body weight, more favorable fat distribution, and fewer menstrual cycles. All this adds up to a 50 percent decreased risk.

Vegetarian Diet

Girls on vegetarian diets have later menarche in many studies. Girls who eat more meat have an earlier menarche.

Soy, But Only with Caution

Dr. Ken Setchell says: "It's probably safe to say that early exposure is best. The earlier the change is made, the greater the long-term benefit is likely to be. The evidence? Look at Asian women who eat soy all through their lives and have lower breast cancer rates throughout their lifetime." However, many researchers are very cautious when it comes to this age group. Sure, large doses could help prevent breast cancer, but excessive amounts of soy in chimps does stunt growth. What parent would be willing to risk a major drop in stature by feeding his or her child a soy-rich diet that is so low in calories that growth is impaired? Can you imagine what scorn your friends would heap on you for keeping your daughter artificially a little girl, when their own daughters were already developing breasts and dating? This could be a hugely humiliating experience for many little girls. It's really a question that society has to ask after much more data is in. In traditional Asian diets, soy makes sense, but for others, the data is just not there yet.

Growth Charts

Clearly, obsessive amounts of exercise and very low-calorie diets will prevent breast cancer, but at what cost in terms of other risks to an adolescent's health? If you are determined to delay your daughter's menarche, it's really critical to follow her growth charts carefully to be certain that you aren't stunting her growth. Her diet would have to be very restrictive and her exercise program very strenuous — that is, near that of an elite-class athlete — to have such an effect.

Recommendation

Consider following all of the above measures with the exception of taking soy, which should be discussed carefully with your pediatrician.

ADOLESCENCE TO FIRST FULL-TERM BIRTH

Breast tissue is at its very greatest risk when it is undergoing its fastest development. DNA damage appears to accumulate most rapidly from menarche to time of first birth, says Harvard's Graham Colditz. Thus, "greater understanding of potential for a diet rich in vitamins including antioxidants deserves prompt attention as this may offer important potential to reduce lifetime risk." Adolescence is the time of greatest vulnerability to any part of the pathways that cause cancer. Cells in the breast are both rapidly dividing and growing. This highly sensitive tissue represents a prime opportunity for genetic mistakes to occur. Too many X rays, exposure to pesticides, cigarette smoke, excess estrogen, and other chemicals all require the maximum amount of "chemoprotection." Breast tissue does not finish its development until a woman has competed a full-term delivery.

Measures That Cut the Estrogen Effect and the Estrogen Pathway

Adolescence continues to be a time when foods that could hurt you should be scrupulously avoided. Those include polyunsaturated fats, transfatty acids, red meats — any foods with the potential for high organochlorine concentrations.

Measures That Protect the Milk Ducts

Eat fruits and vegetables: The key protective factors during this time are diets rich in fruits and vegetables. Antioxidants may be especially needed during a period of rapid cell growth and divisions.

Eat foods that are high in protein: Protein helps breast tissue to mature more quickly, protecting against prolonged exposure to dangerous elements. Eating 20 percent of calories as protein is the recommendation.

Don't smoke: New and convincing evidence finally demonstrates that smoking does increase the risk of breast cancer. One reason the evidence took so long to accumulate is that even girls who were exposed to passive smoke had an increased risk — leaving very few girls exposed to no smoke as a group to which comparisons could be made.

Avoid chemical estrogens: The big worry is that girls, teenagers, and young women are not protected from the chemicals that can affect developing breasts and can store chemical estrogens in their breasts for a lifetime. Although the debate is far from over, I would carefully protect any child from potentially carcinogenic chemicals, including cleaning products and pesticides used for rodents, insects, and bees. Pay careful attention to posted warnings at schools, playgrounds, and other locations when pesticides are in use. Avoid food that may have high quantities of chemical estrogens.

Consider soy: The allure of soy is that it may mature breast ducts earlier, making them more immune to the effects of harmful cancer-causing substances. That's certainly been proven in animal studies. For instance, genistein matures the breast duct cells in prepubescent rats, so the potential of cells to become cancerous is minimized. Some researchers conclude that early genistein consumption is essential for protection against adult breast cancer.

However, says Dr. Anna Wu of USC, it is still to be determined if there could be any harmful effects in eating soy at a young age. Clearly, over a billion Asian women eat soy their entire lives without any known risks. Yet laboratory experiments show that soy at this age may also cause duct cell proliferation. Until it is known whether or not that is harmful, most scientists are adopting a wait-and-see attitude. The chances are excellent that FDA-approved chemoprevention strategies will be well worked out before your teenager is at risk of contracting breast cancer, making soy less of an imperative.

Warning: Genistein supplements should be strictly avoided. While natural soy foods may have a real protective advantage, genistein taken alone may spur growth in breast cells.

Recommendation

Intergenerational breast cancer prevention is such a new field that the rules haven't even been contemplated yet. I heartily recommend all those measures that fall in line with rigorous good health to help your daughters prevent breast cancer the best way possible, with early intervention. Diets too high in calories are the major danger. The use of soy needs to be discussed with your pediatrician. Remember that just because a cancer runs in a family does not mean that cancer genes are involved. Children may be exposed to the same environmental hazards and the same poor diet and lack of exercise that put their mothers at risk for cancer.

HEALTHY

CUISINES

The foods of the breast cancer prevention diet are only raw ingredients. Hundreds of millions of women around the world suffer a risk of breast cancer that is minuscule compared to Americans'. They transform the foods of the breast cancer prevention diet into spectacular cuisines. That transformation has developed into a fine art over thousands of years of experimentation with herbs, spices, and food ingredients. Scientists who study these cultures and their risk of disease know that they are observing a finely controlled experiment . . . far better than any they could construct. These cultures have stable populations who have eaten the same foods for centuries. That means researchers can be sure these populations are really eating the foods they say they are eating, and they can also be certain that the low rates of breast cancer they observe really can be traced to the foods they eat. What they are learning is that healthy cuisines are the perfect solution — foods with a perfect track record embedded in cuisines that are pleasing to the palate. In my other books I've looked at dozens of different cultures and diets. When it comes to preventing breast cancer, there are really just two cuisines that have demonstrated effectiveness: the Asian diet and the Mediterranean.

THE ASIAN DIET

The Asian diet delivers the lowest breast cancer rates on earth. Oldways Preservation and Exchange Trust, a nonprofit food and nutrition education organization, gained international recognition for identifying cultures that offer healthy, appetizing ways to eat. Their newest project is the Asian diet, based on observations of dietary patterns in South and East Asia, from Indonesia to Korea and along the Pacific rim. Let's look at how the Asian diet incorporates nearly every one of the principles of a breast cancer prevention diet.

The Asian diet is the ultimate low-fat diet. Only 14 percent of the calories eaten by the Chinese come from fat, as compared to about 34 to 43 percent of calories eaten by Americans. The Chinese average only 34 grams of fat a day. But this low-fat diet is one that really works. Most Americans on a low-fat diet gain large amounts of weight. On an Asian diet, you truly can eat more to weigh less. That's because leanness is directly related to the composition of the diet. Why? A plant-based diet that is low in fat, low in animal protein, and high in fiber burns off more calories as body heat. In fact the world's leanest peoples (who are healthy and not starving), based on height, weight, and skin-fold measurements, are the Koreans and

Japanese, according to anthropologist Stephen Bailey, Ph.D., of Tufts University. How is it possible to be so lean? Fiber is one of the Asians' biggest secrets, keeping them full and satisfied with fiber, not calories. In contrast to Americans' meager 10 grams, the Chinese average 77 grams of fiber a day. The proper Chinese diet is also a low-glucose-load diet. Ironically, in 1974 both the developed and the developing world ate roughly the same amount of carbohydrates, 1,680 calories per day, but the kinds of carbohydrates were strikingly different. In the developing world, 98 percent of the carbos were made from cereals, roots, and other staples. In the developed world, only 62 percent came from those healthful foods; the rest came from fruits and sugars. Those extra calories were enough to do enormous damage. The Asian diet is also responsible for the world's longest-lived peoples. Local officials on Okinawa have kept records for over 115 years and can document that the island has more centenarians than any other country. Walk through the villages. You'll be struck that, at 8 or 98, everyone remains lean and taut. You'll see six generations all living together, with the oldest still working a full day. Researchers I spoke with in Okinawa credit a spectacular diet rich in fish and "magic" fruits and vegetables that combine incredible taste with spectacular nutrition. The most magic of these foods is soy, which is consumed in large quantities for breakfast, lunch, and dinner. More to the point, the basic ingredients of the Asian diet all add up to the world's lowest rates of breast cancer.

Plant food is the core of the daily intake in the traditional

Asian diet. Common plant foods include rice and other grains, noodles, flatbreads, potatoes, fruits, vegetables — including sea vegetables — nuts, seeds, beans, various soy foods, other legumes, vegetable and nut oils, herbs and spices, and plant-based beverages including tea, wine, and beer. When eaten in sufficient amount this healthy Asian diet provides all of the known essential vitamins, minerals, and fiber, which promote health. The biggest fault in the Asian diet is white rice, which has a high glycemic index, says Walter Willett, M.D., chairman of the nutrition department at the Harvard School of Public Health.

I suggest the following books for excellent suggestions on how to develop an Asian meal plan:

Terrific Pacific Cookbook, by Anya von Bremzen and John Welchman (Workman Publishing, 1995)

China Express, by Nina Simonds (William Morrow, 1993)

Beyond Bok Choy, by Rosa Lo San Ross (Artisan, a division of Workman Publishing, 1996)

Classic Chinese Cuisine, by Nina Simonds (Chapters Publishers & Booksellers, 1994)

Note: The "Meal Plans" chapter of this book lists complete menus using the Asian diet.

THE PREMIER MEDITERRANEAN DIET

A 1948 Rockefeller Foundation study showed that adults living in regions bordering the Mediterranean Sea had the lowest rates of chronic disease in the world. Since then, study after study has shown that women in Mediterranean countries from Spain through Greece come up time and again with low rates of breast cancer. But it is the Greek island of Crete that represents the epitome of the healthy Mediterranean diet.

Nancy Harmon Jenkins, nationally known food writer and author of *The Mediterranean Diet Cookbook,* has long studied the Mediterranean diet. "The Mediterranean diet is so obviously healthy. It is full of fresh vegetables, is high in fiber, and very low in saturated fat. The next best thing is that these foods are familiar to us. It doesn't require us to make great leaps to enjoy the tradition," says Nancy. The true Mediterranean diet also has a low glucose load. Although the Mediterranean diet has been mistaken as the pasta diet, in Crete not a lot of pasta is eaten. That's really more of an American interpretation! The Mediterranean diet, however, is not a low-fat diet. How much fat does it have? According to Oldways Preservation and Exchange Trust, the Mediterranean diet is about 30 percent fat. Annie Copps of Oldways says, "It's even healthy at as high as 40 percent if the person is active and the fat is mostly vegetarian based." In Crete, the fat that is present is mostly in the form of olive oil. The more olive oil, the lower the rate of breast cancer. But there is a real need not to overdo the Mediterranean diet. In the 1960s, when it was a very modest-calorie diet, it boasted the lowest incidence of overall cancer and heart disease in the world. But the Cretans have lost the heart disease edge to the Japanese. What's changed? The Cretans have nearly doubled their animal fat, potato, and egg intake while quadrupling the amount of meat they eat. Where the traditional Cretan diet was virtually all vegetarian, it is now becoming far higher in meat. The bottom line is simple. The vegetarian diet of old, laced with olive oil, is an extremely healthy choice. It is high in complex carbohydrates from grains and legumes, and high in fiber from vegetables and fruit. Fresh plants, cereals, and olive oil secure a high intake of beta-carotene, vitamin C, tocopherols, and minerals. The diet is filled with olive oil, leaves from lettuce, spinach, Swiss chard, pasta, purslane, and many different kinds of vegetables, cheese, fruit, and wine. But as the calories climb, so do the risks. The Cretans of 1960 were indeed lean and fit. The big jump in fat intake and calories has widened their girth. In the next chapter you will find Mediterranean menus prepared by *Mediterranean Diet Cookbook* author Nancy Harmon Jenkins.

Recommendation

Your greatest success in following a breast cancer prevention diet will lie in adopting a cuisine that has successfully protected women for hundreds of years. You have the reassurance that this is a safe diet and that these populations have the lowest breast cancer rates in the world. Eat an Asian diet if you and your doctor agree on an estrogen receptor blocker strategy based on soy. Otherwise, consider a Mediterranean diet.

MEAL PLANS

Americans have grown to view foods in two different ways: first and foremost as recreational drugs, drugs that need to taste delicious and quickly lift our spirits — from potato chips and French fries to hamburgers and pasta. Alternatively, we view foods as bitter medicines to be eaten with nose pinched in an effort to prevent disease or heal ourselves. The following meals uniquely incorporate the principles of "feedforward" eating that will allow you to improve both your mood and hunger control through foods that are both good for you and make you feel terrific.

Feedforward eating means ingesting the foods that will give you the mood and energy level you'd like to have after every meal. That might mean eating more alerting foods in the morning, more calming foods in the afternoon, and more soporific foods in the evening. In other words, choosing in advance exactly how you would want to feel.

Feedforward eating is consuming the right foods in advance of a meeting, a workout, a nap, or concentrated intellectual effort so that you feel and perform exactly as you want. With feedforward eating, you plan your day according to how you want to feel at a given time or for a specific activity. This is fully described in my last book, *Dr. Bob Arnot's Revolutionary Weight Control Program.*

The reason feedforward eating works so well is this: The brains natural craving for foods serves to meet specific needs to make hormones and neurotransmitters, replace spent fuel stores, or rebuild damaged muscle. By the time you crave nutrients to meet those needs, you've already suffered a serious deficiency. The body signals you with urgent warnings that force you to overcorrect, which means overeating, often all of the wrong foods.

In the following meal plans, you'll find lots of fun and interesting examples for breakfast, lunch, and dinner. For each meal there are three separate categories, Asian, Mediterranean, and the New American plan. They were methodically prepared by Nancy Jenkins and by Rita Mitchell and Barbara Sutherland, of the University of California at Berkeley, who carefully included all the components described in the previous chapters. Complete meal plans for breakfast, lunch, and dinner follow brief descriptions of each cuisine.

ASIAN

These meals are rich in soy protein, fiber, and cruciferous vegetables and are low in glucose load and fat. They are the ideal breast cancer prevention meals. They contain whole grains and approximately nine servings of fruits and vegetables a day, including two cruciferous vegetables. They are low in fat and have about 25 to 35 grams of fiber. The Asian menus contain approximately 20 percent of calories as protein, 15 to 20 percent as fat, and 60 to 65 percent as carbohydrates. These meals contain soy products that are very high in genistein, which keeps the total amount of soy protein closer to 35 grams.

These meals are specifically for women before the menopause who want a high soy-based diet.

If you and your doctor are not enthusiastic about soy, you will want to choose meal plans from the Mediterranean or new American cuisines.

Breakfast

SOY SMOOTHIE
soy milk, nonfat milk, banana, calcium-fortified orange juice.
Rice and vegetables.

Tempeh with snow peas, mushrooms, carrots.

PHO
spicy soup of rice noodles, sliced tempeh, fresh bean sprouts, green onions, tomato, onions, fish sauce, coriander.

Brown rice griddle cakes with curried tofu, served with fresh papaya and mango chutney.

Miso soup with brown rice, giant kelp, carrot, mushroom, slivered tofu, scallions.

Lunch

HEARTY TOFU MUSHROOM SOUP

Julienne strips of firm tofu, black mushrooms, button mushrooms, shiitake mushrooms, bok choy, and leeks in vegetable broth seasoned lightly with miso, oyster sauce, and rice wine.

Finishing touch — orange slices in orange water.

MOO SHU VEGETABLE

Wrapped in a moo shu wrapper is the filling of bean sprouts, black mushrooms, shredded carrot, snow peas, cabbage, and onion, garnished with plum sauce and chopped green onions.

Finishing touch — pear-apple slices.

VEGETABLE TOFU LIGHT STIR-FRY

Firm tofu, snow peas, shiitake mushrooms, broccoli, water chestnuts, seasoned with garlic, oil, sherry vinegar, and tamari soy sauce, and served on a bed of brown rice.

Finishing touch — kiwifruit and pear slices.

SWEET AND SOUR TOFU WITH ASPARAGUS AND RADISH SALAD

Tofu and onion in a light sweet and sour sauce served on a bed of brown rice with fresh asparagus, cauliflower, and radishes lightly seasoned with soy sauce, sesame oil, and rice vinegar.

Finishing touch — mandarin orange wedges.

TOFU AND VEGETABLE NOODLES

Lightly stir-fried broccoli, cauliflower, bok choy, black mushrooms, onions, water chestnuts, tofu, and fresh ginger, served over buckwheat noodles, garnished with bamboo shoots and cilantro.

     Finishing touch — banana and dried cranberries.

Dinner

TOFU CURRY

Tofu with tomato, carrots, onion, cauliflower, green beans, seasoned with garlic, ginger, turmeric, coriander, and cumin. Served over brown rice and topped with nonfat plain yogurt.

     Finishing touch — lychees and mango ice.

LAOTIAN FISH SOUP

Freshwater fish, green onions, tomato, carrot, broccoli, fish sauce, lemongrass, lemon juice. Served with a bowl of brown rice.

     Finishing touch — banana baked in orange water.

SWEET AND SOUR TEMPEH

Tempeh with carrots, green peppers, bok choy, onion, pineapple chunks, and ginger in a tangy sweet and sour sauce. Served on a bed of brown rice.

     Finishing touch — homemade lowfat mango sorbet.

GRILLED FRESH TUNA WITH VEGETABLES

Fresh tuna, grilled, served with a stir-fry of broccoli, cauliflower, snow peas, water chestnut, sweet red pepper. Served with brown rice.

> Finishing touch — papaya and strawberries.

STIR-FRY TOFU AND VEGETABLES IN BLACK BEAN SAUCE

A stir-fry of firm tofu, green beans, onions, bok choy, broccoli, mushrooms, carrots, sweet red pepper. Served over a bed of rice noodles.

> Finishing touch — mung bean cake.

MEDITERRANEAN

These menus feature the distinctive flavors of the Mediterranean. They are constructed without soy protein for those women who choose not to employ the estrogen receptor blocker strategy or are allergic to soy or who simply prefer Mediterranean foods. This is a higher-fat diet, with the primary fats being olive oil and fish oil. You'll find approximately nine servings of fruits and vegetables a day, including two cruciferous vegetables. They are moderate in fat, and rich in omega-9 fatty acids. They contain about 25 to 35 grams of fiber. The Mediterranean menus contain approximately 20 percent of calories as protein, 25 to 30 percent as fat, and 50 to 55 percent as carbohydrates.

Breakfast

Lowfat goat cheese with melon and figs. Toasted dense whole wheat bread. Orange juice.

Low-fat artichoke frittata. Grilled Roma tomatoes garnished with fresh basil.

Black olive focaccia. Grapefruit juice.

Sliced fresh peaches and mixed berries, topped with lowfat vanilla yogurt. Corn meal, whole wheat waffles. Pineapple juice.

Buckwheat date crepes topped with orange slices and lowfat vanilla yogurt. Strawberry-guava nectar.

SMOOTHIE
Lowfat vanilla yogurt, peaches, fresh orange. Toasted whole wheat nut bread.

Lunch

PITA BREAD SANDWICH
A whole wheat pita bread filled with hummus and sweet red peppers, topped with chopped black olives, Italian parsley, and nonfat plain yogurt.

Finishing touch — Fuji apple slices and figs.

HEARTY MINESTRONE

Potato, carrots, celery, onion, cabbage, French beans, Italian tomato, spinach, haricot beans, garbanzo beans, and kidney beans in vegetable broth topped with a light sprinkle of fresh grated Romano cheese. Served with whole wheat focaccia.

Finishing touch — Bosc pear slices.

SPRING CRACKED WHEAT SALAD

Asparagus, mushrooms, Italian tomatoes, red onions, dressed lightly with olive oil and balsamic vinegar, served on a bed of cracked wheat and garnished with Italian parsley. Served with whole wheat bread sticks.

Finishing touch — sliced kiwifruit and banana.

GREEK SANDWICH

Seven-grain bread, brushed with olive oil, filled with pears, walnuts, romaine lettuce, and crumbled feta. Served with broccoli salad.

Finishing touch — strawberries.

MEDLEY SALAD

Eggplant, red, yellow, and green sweet peppers, zucchini, green onions, cauliflower, lightly tossed in a yogurt–garlic dressing, garnished with raisins. Served with a whole wheat roll.

Finishing touch — plums.

Dinners

VEGETABLE AND BEAN RAGOUT OVER COUSCOUS

Garbanzo beans, potato, tomato, onion, red pepper, and kale, seasoned with coriander, cinnamon, lemon, saffron. Served over couscous. Field greens with light vinaigrette.

Finishing touch — apple and grapefruit slices with currants.

GREEN CABBAGE STUFFED WITH BULGUR AND VEGETABLES

Cabbage leaves, bulgur, mushrooms, roasted butternut squash, onion, and raisins, seasoned with nutmeg, served with lowfat plain yogurt. Baked tomato. Dense whole wheat roll.

Finishing touch — fresh strawberries with lemon sorbet.

BOUILLABAISSE

Variety of fish, onion, tomato, sweet red pepper, broccoli, navy beans, seasoned with garlic, basil, saffron. Served with hearty whole wheat bread. Romaine with light vinaigrette.

Finishing touch — mixed berry ice.

RATATOUILLE

A robust casserole of eggplant, onion, green pepper, zucchini, tomato, kale, sautéed in olive oil, topped with a sprinkle of

fresh grated Romano cheese. Served with whole wheat
French bread. Spinach salad with orange dressing.

> Finishing touch — minted melon slices.

LINGUINE WITH LENTILS

Buckwheat linguine with lentils, eggplant, carrot, onion, and
chard, dusted with freshly grated parmesan cheese. Served
with fresh sliced Roma tomatoes dressed lightly with olive oil.
Hearty whole wheat bread.

> Finishing touch — plums with nonfat yogurt.

NEW AMERICAN

These menus have a mix of Asian and American foods, yet are
still rich in legumes and whole grains, high in fiber, and low in
glucose load. The New American menus contain approximately nine servings of fruits and vegetables a day, including
two cruciferous vegetables. They have from 25 to 35 grams of
fiber. The New American menus contain approximately 20 percent of calories as protein, 20 percent as fat, and 60 percent as
carbohydrates. You're likely to find most of these foods at your
local grocery store.

Breakfast

Homemade muesli, lowfat plain yogurt. Orange slices.
Grapefruit juice.

Coarse-cut oatmeal sprinkled with bran, sun-dried cranberries, and walnuts, served with nonfat milk. Orange juice.

EGGS FLORENTINE
Poached eggs served on a bed of wilted spinach, coated with a lowfat sauce, dusted with freshly grated parmesan cheese. Served with toasted hearty whole wheat bread. Apple-cranberry juice.

Dense, grainy, buckwheat pancakes laden with fresh berries and juice. Served with a glass of nonfat milk. Mango-guava nectar.

All bran cereal with soy milk and banana. Pineapple juice.

Lunch

VEGETABLE-POTATO SALAD
Potato, carrots, asparagus, shredded red cabbage, Fuji apple, red onion, parsley, on a bed of Belgian endive, lightly dressed with olive oil and balsamic vinegar. Served with a whole wheat sesame-seed roll.
Finishing touch — kiwifruit.

BURRITO
Whole wheat tortilla filled with black beans, brown rice, broccoli flowerets, green onion, small amount lowfat white

cheddar cheese, seasoned with fresh tomato-corn salsa and cilantro.

Finishing touch — strawberry and orange fruit plate.

CUCUMBER-WALNUT SOUP

Cucumber, green onions, kale, nonfat plain yogurt, walnuts, seasoned with dill, garlic. Served with whole wheat bran roll.

Finishing touch — lemon-raspberry sorbet.

OPEN-FACE SANDWICH

Lentil-nut loaf topped with sun-dried tomatoes and a sprinkle of chopped green onion, served warm on a whole wheat baguette with a fresh spinach and red cabbage salad, dressed lightly with a tangy tofu dressing.

Finishing touch — dried fig slices and nonfat vanilla yogurt.

SPRING SALAD

Baby artichoke hearts, sweet red pepper, cauliflower, mushrooms, green peas on a bed of brown rice, garnished with a light sprinkle of roasted sesame seeds and dressed with olive oil and balsamic vinegar. Served with Ak-Mak whole wheat crackers.

Finishing touch — Mandarin orange wedges.

Dinner

BLACK BEAN AND MUSHROOM STEW WITH POLENTA

Black beans and mushroom ragout with parmesan polenta. Served with salad of arugula, butter lettuce, radicchio, shredded red cabbage, dressed with a little olive oil and lemon juice.

Finishing touch — peach slices and raspberries served with lemon sherbet.

GRILLED SWORDFISH

Swordfish brushed with olive oil and grilled, garnished with roasted corn and red pepper salsa. Served with quinoa, kale, carrots, and a whole wheat roll.

Finishing touch — ginger yogurt.

THREE-BEAN CHILI

Spicy chili made with a mix of three beans (red, garbanzo, and cranberry), onion, celery, kale and red chili. Served with whole wheat tortillas. Mixed greens and tomato with light vinaigrette.

Finishing touch — honeydew melon and blueberries.

BLACK BEAN AND RICE SOUP

A hearty soup of black beans, brown rice, and vegetables, served with whole wheat bread and a spinach and orange salad tossed in olive oil and balsamic vinegar.

Finishing touch — fresh figs, walnuts, and honey garnished with whipped vanilla cream cheese.

STUFFED RED PEPPERS
Large red peppers stuffed with brown rice, wild rice, broccoli flowerets, green onion, and raisins, topped with lowfat cheddar cheese and served with a side of asparagus. Grainy whole wheat roll.

Finishing touch — poached apple with almond and walnuts topped with lowfat vanilla yogurt.

Alternatively, you may plan your own meals from the foods and tables listed in the previous chapters. That's what we've done at home, simply incorporating the foods of the breast cancer prevention diet into our own meals. I'd suggest finding ten new meals to replace your ten favorite meals of today. Once you've mastered them, you'll then find eating the breast cancer prevention diet easy and fun, without the need to struggle with new shopping lists. You'll want to stick with just one cuisine rather than mixing and matching, since all of the nutrient values have been calculated for an entire day of eating the foods of just one cuisine.

SUPPLEMENTS

A schedule for supplements is listed for breakfast, lunch, and dinner, showing how the doses of fish oil, soy, and indole-3 carbinol should be divided. At the end of the day, you'll find that you've taken 10 grams of fish oil, 60 grams of soy protein, and 500 milligrams of indole-3 carbinol. You may choose to take some or all of these supplements, in consultation with your physician.

Breakfast

Fish oil: Three (1-gram) capsules
Soy shake: 20 grams
or
Flaxseed: 9 grams

Lunch

Indole-3 carbinol: 500 milligrams
Fish oil: three (1-gram) capsules
Soy shake: 20 grams
or
Flaxseed: 9 grams

Dinner

Fish oil: four (1-gram) capsules
Soy shake: 20 grams
or
Flaxseed: 9 grams

CLOSE

We are entering a new era when breast cancer can and will be prevented. Over the next five years we will see spectacular results from the use of preventive drugs such as raloxifene and aromatase inhibitors for women at high risk. These prove that blocking the estrogen effect really works. But many women would rather use diet than drugs to prevent breast cancer. Others will want to add a drug's benefit to dietary adjustments.

As set out at the beginning of this book, there is an extraordinary bet to be made, a bet that diet can strikingly alter your odds of developing breast cancer. An international race of great intensity is now under way to prove once and for all what every component of the breast cancer prevention diet would be. This is no frivolous exercise. Millions are being spent by governments, foundations, and institutions on the breast cancer prevention diet. You can wait a decade or longer for the final results. Or you can act now on an educated guess based on research at the finest institutions in the world. It's a bet that thousands of breast cancer survivors are already making and billions of other women around the world have already made — that diet can prevent cancer.

"I really believe in this diet," says Deborah McCurdy. "I believe it's going to keep me cancer-free and healthy and help my family from getting sick. I don't want them to have to go through what I did. I believe so strongly in this diet, in this way of eating, that when I developed pneumonia after my bone marrow transplant, and I was in the hospital, I insisted on staying with the plan and the hospital went along with me — they let my family bring in fresh fruits and vegetables and my soy drinks, and the hospital prepared meals that fit into the diet. I was so motivated that even with pneumonia, I wanted to keep on eating right. I really didn't want to cheat, because I was enjoying what I was eating. And I didn't cheat, because I really believe in it."

We're making that bet in our home, and we hope you will too.

Appendix: Genistein Values

This table shows how much genistein you get in 100 grams (roughly three and a half ounces, or a little less than a quarter of a pound) of soy-based foods.

Food	Genistein Mg/100 gram
Soy flakes, defatted	195
Soy flakes	156
Soy flakes, full fat	132
Soy flakes, defatted, toasted	105
Soybean meal, whole	100
Soy flour	94
Soy nuts	94
Soy concentrate, water extracted	91
Soybeans, roasted	87
Soy flour, defatted	75
Soy granule	75

Food	Genistein Mg/100 gram
Soybeans, green	73
Soy protein, textured	71
Soybeans, dried	70
Soy flour, defatted, dried	60
Soy milk powder	57
Soy isolate	56
Miso	52
Tofu, dry spiced	42
Tempeh	40
Miso paste	38
Akamiso soup mix	37
Shiromiso soup mix	34
Miso (barley)	34
Soy sprouts, Amsoy (5 days)	33
Tofu, Kikkoman firm	31
Soybean paste	30
Soybean chips	28
Soy isolate, acid	27
Miso (rice)	26
Miso paste (rice or barley)	26
Soybean sprouts	23
Soybean sprouts, commercial	23
Soybean curd, fermented	22
Tofu, Azumaya soft	22
Soy concentrate, alcohol extracted	21
Soy fiber	21

Appendix: Genistein Values

Food	Genistein Mg/100 gram
Tofu, Vitasoy-silken	21
Soybeans, dry, whole	20
Tempeh burger	20
Soybean paste/wheat	19
Tofu, Nasoya soft	19
Tofu, Tree of Life	19
Tofu, Mori-Ny	18
Honzukuri miso (rice and soybeans)	18
Tofu	17
Soybean paste/rice	15
Soybean sprouts, homemade (7 days)	11
Soy milk	10
Tofu yogurt	9
Tofu, Weber	9
Soy hot dog	8
Soy bacon	7
Tofu, soft	5
Tofu, hard	5
Soy milk, Banyan	4
Soy cheddar cheese	4
Tofu, fermented	4
Ice bean	4
Soy mozzarella cheese	4
Soy milk, Plum Flower	3
Soy milk	3
Soy milk formula, Isomil	2

The Breast Cancer Prevention Diet

Food	Genistein Mg/100 gram
Soy drink, First Alternative	2
Soy milk formula, ProSobee	2
Soybean paste, hot	2
Soy cheese	2
Tofutti	2
Soy concentrate	1
Soy sauce	1
Soy parmesan	1
Soy-based specialty formula, Enrich	1
Soy-based specialty formula, Jevity	1
Soy-based specialty formula	0
Soybean paste, sweet	0
Soy-based specialty formula, Glucerna	0

Adapted from Nutrition and Cancer *26 (1996):123–148.*

Selected References

Nearly 3,000 scientific studies were reviewed for this book. While there isn't room to include all of them here, I have included some of the most useful and interesting.

ARTICLES

Introduction

Bernstein, L.
Prospects for primary prevention of breast cancer.
American Journal of Epidemiology 135, no. 2 (1992).

Chen, J.
Antioxidant status and cancer mortality in China.
International Journal of Epidemiology (1992).

Ellrod, Gray, et al.
Evidence-based disease management.
Journal of the American Medical Association 278, no. 20 (1997): 1687–1692.

Giovannucci, Edward.
A comparison of prospective and retrospective assessments of diet in the study of breast cancer.
American Journal of Epidemiology 137, no. 5 (1993).

Lee, H. P., et al.
Dietary effects on breast cancer risk in Singapore.
Lancet 337, no. 8751 (1991): 1197–1200.

Rose, David.
The mechanistic rationale in support of dietary cancer prevention.
Preventive Medicine 25 (1996): 34–37.

Wang, D. Y.
Serum hormone levels in British and rural Chinese females.
Breast Cancer Research and Treatment 188 (1991): S41–S45.

What Makes Breast Cancer Grow

Aldercreutz, Herman, et al.
Diet and plasma androgens in postmenopausal vegetarian and omnivorous women and postmenopausal women with breast cancer.
American Journal of Clinical Nutrition 49 (1989): 442–443.

E2 regulates sst2 expression in breast cell lines through the ER.
Cancer Research 56 (1996): 3655–3658.

Hartmann, Arndt.
Molecular epidemiology of P53 gene mutations in human breast cancer.
Trends in Genetics 13 (1997): 27–33.

————. Novel pattern of P53 mutation in breast cancer from Austrian women.
Journal of Clinical Investigation 95 (1995): 686–689.

Hulka, Barbara S., and Azadeh T. Stark.
Breast cancer: cause and prevention.
Lancet 346, no. 8979 (1995): 883.

Planas-Silva, Maricarmen D., and Robert A. Weinberg.
Estrogen-dependent cyclin E-cdk2 activation through P21 redistribution.
Molecular and Cellular Biology 17, no. 7 (1997): 4059–4069.

Rose, David P.
Diet, hormones and cancer.
Annual Review of Public Health 14 (1993): 1–18.

Saitoh, S., et al.
P53 gene mutations in breast cancers in midwestern US women.
Oncogene 9 (1994): 2869–2875.

Shattuck-Eidens, Donna.
BRCA1 sequence analysis in women at high risk for susceptibility mutations.
Journal of the American Medical Association 278, no. 15 (1997): 1242.

Talamini, R.
Special medical conditions and risk of breast cancer.
British Journal of Cancer 75, no. 11 (1997): 1699–1703.

How Foods Can Prevent Breast Cancer

Arpels, John C.
The female brain hypoestrogenic continuum from the premenstrual syndrome to menopause.
Journal of Reproductive Medicine 41, no. 9 (1996).

Bernstein, Leslie.
Endogenous hormones and breast cancer risk.
Epidemiologic Reviews 15, no. 1 (1993).

———. Estrogen and sex hormone binding globulin levels in nulliparous and parous women.
Journal of the National Cancer Institute 74, no. 4 (1985): 741–745.

———. Treatment with human chorionic gonadotropin and risk of breast cancer.
Cancer Epidemiology, Biomarkers and Prevention 4 (1995): 437–440.

Breast cancer and hormone replacement therapy: collaborative re-analysis of data from 51 epidemiological studies of 52,705 women with breast cancer and 108,411 women without breast cancer.
Collaborative Group on Hormonal Factors in Breast Cancer 350, no. 9084 (1997).

Catalano, M.G., et al.
Sex steroid binding protein receptor is related to a reduced proliferation rate in human breast cancer.
Breast Cancer Research and Treatment 42, no. 3 (1997): 227–234.

Selected References

El-Tanani, M. K. K., and C. D. Green
Interaction between estradiol and growth factors in the regulation
of specific gene expression in MCF-7 human breast cancer cells.
Journal of Steroid Biochemistry and Molecular Biology 60, nos. 5–6
(1996): 269–276.

Gorbach, Sherwood L.
Diet and the excretion and enterohepatic cycling of estrogens.
Preventive Medicine 16 (1987): 525–531.

Nananda, F.
Patient specific decisions about hormone replacement therapy in
post-menopausal women.
Journal of the American Medicine Association 277, no. 14 (1997).

Prentice, Ross.
Dietary fat reduction and plasma estradiol concentration in healthy
post-menopausal women.
Journal of the National Cancer Institute 82, no. 2 (1990).

A prospective study of endogenous estrogens and breast cancer in
postmenopausal women.
Journal of the National Cancer Institute 87, no. 3 (1995): 190–197.

Sherwin, Barbara B.
Estrogen effects on cognition in menopausal women.
Neurology 48, suppl. 7 (1997).

Shimizu, H.
Serum estrogen levels in postmenopausal women: comparison of
American whites and Japanese in Japan.
British Journal of Cancer 61 (1990): 421–433.

Sonnenschein, C.
Development of a marker of estrogenic exposure in human serum.
Clinical Chemistry 41 (December 1996): 1888–1895.

Trichopoulos, D.
The effect of westernization on urine estrogens, frequency of ovulation and breast cancer risk.
Cancer 53, no. 1 (1984): 187–192.

Woods, Margo N.
Hormonal levels during dietary changes in premenopausal African American women.
Journal of the National Cancer Institute 88, no. 19 (1996): 1369–1374.

Zava, D. T.
Estrogenic activity of natural and synthetic estrogens in human breast cancer cells in culture.
Environmental Health Perspectives 105 (April 1997): 637–645.

Step 1: Block the Estrogen Receptor

Aldercreutz, C. H.
Soybean phytoestrogen intake and cancer risk.
Journal of Nutrition 125, no. 3 (1995): 757S–770S.

Anderson, James W.
Meta-analysis of the effects of soy protein intake on serum lipids.
New England Journal of Medicine 333, no. 5 (1995): 276–282.

Selected References

Barnes, S.
Rationale for the use of genistein containing soy matrices in chemo-
prevention trials for breast and prostate cancer.
Journal of Cellular Biochemistry 22 (1995): 181–187.

Barnes, Stephen.
Soy isoflavonoids and cancer prevention. In *Dietary Phytochemicals
in Cancer Prevention and Treatment.* American Institute for Cancer
Research, ed.
New York: Plenum Press, 1996.

Cassidy, Aedin, and Sheila Bingham.
Biological effects of isoflavones in young women.
British Journal of Nutrition 74, no. 4 (1995): 587–601.

Cassidy, Aedin, Sheila Bingham, and K. D. R. Setchell.
Biological effects of a diet of soy protein rich in isoflavones on the
menstrual cycle of premenopausal women.
American Journal of Clinical Nutrition 60, no. 3 (1994): 333–340.

Coward, Lori.
Genistein, daidzein and their beta-glycoside conjugates.
Journal of Agricultural and Food Chemistry 41 (1993).

Eastman, P.
Phytamins are not ready for public consumption.
Journal of the National Cancer Institute 87 (1995): 1430–1432.

Ingram, David, et al.
Case-control study of phyto-estrogens and breast cancer.
Lancet 350, no. 9083 (1997): 990–994.

Jacobs, Maryce M.
Potential role of dietary isoflavones in the prevention of cancer.
In M.M. Jacobs, ed., *Diet and Cancer.* New York: Plenum Press,
1994.

Kennedy, A. R.
The evidence for soybean products as cancer preventive agents.
Journal of Nutrition 125, no. 3 (1995): 733S–743S.

Kurzer, Mindy S., and Xia Xu.
Dietary phytoestrogens.
Annual Review of Nutrition 17 (1997): 353–381.

Lamartiniere, Coral A., et al.
Genistein suppresses mammary cancer in rats.
Carcinogenesis 16, no. 111 (1995): 2833–2840.

Martin, M. E.
Interactions between phytoestrogens and human sex steroid binding
protein.
Life Sciences 58, no. 5 (1996): 429–436.

Messina, Mark J.
Soy intake and cancer risk.
Nutrition and Cancer 21, no. 2 (1994): 113–131.

Molteni, A.
In vitro hormonal effects of soybean isoflavones.
Journal of Nutrition 125, no. 3 (1995): 751S–756S.

Nesbitt, Paula D., and Lilian U. Thompson.
Lignans in homemade and commercial products containing flaxseed.
Nutrition and Cancer 29, no. 3 (1997): 222–227.

Peterson, Greg, and Stephen Barnes
Genistein inhibits both estrogen and growth factor–stimulated proliferation of human breast cancer cells.
Cell Growth and Differentiation 7, no. 10 (1996): 1345–1351.

Peterson, T. Greg, et al.
The role of metabolism in mammary epithelial cell growth inhibition by the isoflavones genistein and biochanin A.
Carcinogenesis 17, no. 9 (1996): 1861–1869.

Reinli, K.
Phytoestrogen content of foods.
Nutrition and Cancer 26, no. 2 (1996): 123–148.

Setchell, K. D. R.
Dietary estrogens — a probable cause of infertility and liver disease in captive cheetahs.
Gastroenterology 93 (1987): 225–233.

———. Exposure of infants to phyto estrogens from soy-based infant formula.
Lancet 349, no. 9070 (1997): 23–27.

———. Lignans in man and in animal species.
Nature 288, no. 5784 (1980): 740–742.

————. Natural occurring non-steroidal estrogens of dietary origin. In *Estrogens in the Environment II,* John A. McLachlan, ed. New York: Elsevier Science, 1985.

————. Nonsteroidal estrogens of dietary origin. *American Journal of Clinical Nutrition* 40 (1984): 5569–5578.

————. Nonsteroidal estrogens of dietary origin. *Proceedings of the Nutrition Society of New Zealand* 20 (1995): 1–20.

Thompson, Lilian U., et. al
Antitumorigenic effect of a mammalian lignan precursor from flaxseed.
Nutrition and Cancer 26, no. 2 (1996): 159–165.

————. Flaxseed and its lignan and oil components reduce mammary tumor growth at a late stage of carcinogenesis. *Carcinogenesis* 17, no. 6 (1996):1373.

Verma, S. P.
Curcumin and genistein, plant natural products show synergistic inhibitory effects on the growth of human breast cancer MCF-7 cells induced by estrogenic pesticides. *Biochemical and Biophysical Communications* 233 (1997): 692–696.

Wang, Huei-ju, and Patricia Murphy.
Isoflavone content in commercial soybean foods, *Journal of Agricultural and Food Chemistry* 42, no. 8 (1994): 1666–1673.

Wang, T. T. Y., N. Sathyamoorty, and J. M. Phang.
Molecular effects of genistein on estrogen receptor mediated pathways.
Carcinogenesis 17, no. 2 (1996): 271–275.

Xu, X.
Bioavailability of soybean isoflavones depends upon gut microflora in women.
Journal of Nutrition 125, no. 9 (1995): 2307–2315.

Zajchowski, Deborah A., Ruth Sager, and Lynn Webster
Estrogen inhibits the growth of estrogen receptor–negative, but not estrogen receptor–positive, human mammary epithelial cells expressing a recombinant estrogen receptor.
Cancer Research 53, no. 20 (1993): 5004–5011.

Zava, D. T.
Estrogenic and anti-proliferative properties of genistein and other flavonoids in human breast cancer cells in vitro.
Nutrition and Cancer 27, no. 1 (1997): 31–40.

Zeigler, Regina G.
Quantifying estrogen metabolism.
Environmental Health Perspectives 105, suppl. 3 (1997).

Step 2: Change Fats

Bagga, D.
Dietary modulation of omega-3/omega-6 polyunsaturated fatty acid ratios in patients with breast cancer.
Journal of the National Cancer Institute 89, no. 15 (1997): 1123–1131.

Byers, Tim, Cheryl Rock, and Katherine Hamilton.
Dietary changes after breast cancer.
Cancer Practice 5, no 5. (1997).

Canadian Diet and Breast Cancer Prevention Study Group. Effects
at two years of a low-fat, high-carbohydrate diet on radiologic
features of the breast: results from a randomized trial.
Journal of the National Cancer Institute 8 (1997): 488–496.

Cave, William T., Jr.
Dietary omega-3 polyunsaturated fats and breast cancer.
Nutrition 12, no. 1 (1996): S39–S42.

————— . Omega 3 polyunsaturated fatty acids in rodent models of
breast cancer.
Breast Cancer Research and Treatment 46 (1997).

Caygill, C. P.
Fat, fish, fish oil and cancer.
British Journal of Cancer 74, no. 1 (1996): 159–164.

Cunningham, D. C., L. Y. Harrison, and T. D. Shultz.
Proliferative responses of normal human mammary and MCF-7
breast cancer cells to linoleic acid, conjugated linoleic acid and
eicosanoid synthesis inhibitors in culture.
Anticancer Research 17, no. 1A (1997): 193–203.

Fay, Michael P.
Effect of different types and amounts of fat on the development of
mammary tumors in rodents.
Cancer Research 57 (1997): 3979–3988.

Selected References

Giovannucci, E.
Epidemiologic status of fat and breast cancer.
Cerin Symposium/Nutrition and Cancer.

Godley, P. A.
Essential fatty acid consumption and risk of breast cancer.
Breast Cancer Research and Treatment 35, no. 1 (1995): 91–95.

Johanning, G. L.
Modulation of breast cancer cell adhesion by unsaturated fatty
acids.
Nutrition 12, no. 11–12 (1996): 810–816.

Kilgore, Michael, et al.
MCF-7 and T47D human breast cancer cells contain a functional
peroxisomal response.
Molecular and Cellular Endocrinology 129 , no. 2 (1997): 229–235.

Kohlmeier, Lenore, and Michelle Mendez..
Controversies surrounding diet and breast cancer.
Proceedings of the Nutrition Society 56, no. 1/B (1997): 369–382.

Low-fat, high-fiber diet and serum estrone sulfate in premenopausal women.
American Journal of Clinical Nutrition 49 (1989): 1179–1183.

Petrek, J. A.
Breast cancer risk and fatty acids in the breast and abdominal adi-
pose tissues.
Journal of the National Cancer Institute 86, no. 1 (1994): 53–56.

Rose, David.
Dietary fat, fatty acids and breast cancer.
Breast Cancer 4, no. 1 (1997).

————. Influence of diets containing eicosapentanoic or docosa-hexaenoic acid on growth and metastasis of breast cancer cells in nude mice.
Journal of the National Cancer Institute 877, no. 8 (1995).

Rose, David P.
Dietary fatty acids and cancer.
American Journal of Clinical Nutrition 66 (1997): 998S–1003S.

Simopoulos, Artemis P.
Omega 3 fatty acids in health and disease and in growth and development.
American Journal of Clinical Nutrition 54 (1991): 428–463.

————. Omega 3 fatty acids in growth and development. In *Encyclopedia of Human Biology,* 2d ed., 1997, vol. 6, 409–419.

Tang, Dean G.
Arachidonate piosygensases as essential regulators of cell survival and apoptosis.
Proceedings of the National Academy of Sciences 93 (1996): 5241–5246.

————. Suppression of W256 carcinosarcoma cell apoptosis by arachidonic acid and other polyunsaturated fats.
International Journal of Cancer 72 (1997): 1078–1087.

Weisburger, John H.
Dietary fat and risk of chronic disease.
Journal of the American Dietetic Association 97, no. 7 (1997):
S16–S23.

Wynder, Ernst L.
Breast cancer: weighing the evidence for a promoting role of dietary
fat.
Journal of the National Cancer Institute 89, no. 11 (1997).

Step 3: Make Good Estrogens

Bradlow, H. Leon, et al.
Indole-3 carbinol: a novel approach to breast cancer prevention.
Annals of the New York Academy of Sciences 768 (1996).

———— . 2 hydroxyesterone, the good estrogen.
Journal of Endocrinology 150 (1996): S259–S265.

Dwivedy, I.
Synthesis and characterization of estrogen 2,3 and 3,43 quinones.
Chemical Research in Toxicology 4 (1992): 828–833.

Grubbs, C. J. Chemoprevention of chemically induced mammary
carcinogenesis by indole-3 carbinol. *Anticancer Research* 15, no. 3
(1995): 709–716.

Nebert, D. W.
Elevated estrogen 16 alpha hydroxylase.
Journal of the National Cancer Institute 85, no. 23 (1993):
1888–1891.

Sepkovic, Daniel W.
Catechol estrogen production in rat microsomes after treatment
with indole-3 carbinol.
Steroids 59 (1994).

Wall, Monroe E.
Indoles in edible members of the cruciferae.
Journal of Natural Products 51, no. 1 (1988): 129–135.

Step 4: Lower Insulin; Step 5: Drop Glucose Load

Clayton, S. J., F. E. B. May, and B. R. Westley
Insulin-like growth factors control the regulation of estrogen and
progesterone receptor expression by estrogens.
Molecular and Cellular Endocrinology 128, no. 1–2 (1997): 57–68.

Kaaks, R.
Nutrition, hormones and breast cancer: is insulin the missing link?
Cancer Causes and Control 6 (1996): 605–625.

Step 6: Increase Fiber

Rose, David P.
Dietary fiber, phytoestrogens, and breast cancer. *Nutrition* 8, no. 1
(1992):47–51.

———. Effects of diet supplement with wheat bran on serum estrogen levels in the follicular and luteal phases of the menstrual cycle.
Nutrition 13, no. 6 (1997).

Rose, D. P., et al.
High-fiber diet reduces serum estrogen concentrations in pre-
menopausal women.
American Journal of Clinical Nutrition 54, no. 3 (1991): 520–525.

Tew, B. Y.
A diet high in wheat fiber decreases the bioavailability of soybean
isoflavones in a single meal fed to women.
Journal of Nutrition 126, no. 4 (1996): 871–877.

Step 7: Lower Oxidative Load

Djuric, Zora, et al.
Levels of 5-hydroxymethyl-2-deoxyuridine in DNA from blood as a
marker of breast cancer.
Cancer 77, no. 4 (1996): 691–696.

Drewnowski, Adam, and Cheryl L. Rock.
The influence of genetic taste markers on food acceptance.
American Journal of Clinical Nutrition 62 (1995): 506–511.

Franceschi, Silvia, et al.
Intake of micronutrients and risk of breast cancer
Lancet 347, no. 9012 (1996) 1351–1356.

Gerster, H.
The potential role of lycopene for human health.
Journal of the American College of Nutrition 16, no. 2 (1997):
109–126.

Pierce, John P.
Feasibility of a randomized trial of high vegetable diet to prevent
breast cancer recurrence.
Nutrition and Cancer 28, no. 3 (1997): 282–288.

Rock, Cheryl L.
Responsiveness of carotenoids to a high vegetable diet intervention designed to prevent breast cancer recurrence.
Cancer Epidemiology, Biomarkers and Prevention 6 (August 1997): 617–623.

Step 8: Avoid Chemical Estrogens

Bernstein, L.
Serum hormone levels in pre-menopausal Chinese women in Shanghai and white women in Los Angeles.
Cancer Causes and Control 1 (1990): 51–58.

Bradlow, H. L.
Effects of pesticides on the ratio of 16 alpha/2-hydroxyestrone.
Environmental Health Perspectives (1995): 147–150.

Hunter, D. J.
Plasma organochlorine levels and the risk of breast cancer. *New England Journal of Medicine* (1997): 1253–1258.

Shekhar, P .V .M.
Environmental estrogen stimulation of growth and estrogen receptor function in preneoplastic and cancerous human breast cell lines.
Journal of the National Cancer Institute 89, no. 23 (1997).

vant Veer, Pieter.
DDT dicophane and postmenopausal breast cancer in Europe.
British Medical Journal 314, no. 7100 (1997): 81.

Wolff, M. S.
Blood levels of organochlorine residues and risk of breast cancer.
Journal of the National Cancer Institute 85, no. 8 (1993): 648–652.

————. Breast cancer and environmental risk factors.
Annual Review of Pharmacology and Toxicology 36 (1996):
573–596.

Step 9: Decrease Body Fat

Bernstein, L.
Physical exercise and reduced risk of breast cancer in young women.
Journal of the National Cancer Institute 86, no. 18 (1994).

Gammon, Marilie D., Esther M. John, and Julie A. Britton.
Recreational and occupational physical activities and risk of breast
cancer. *Journal of the National Cancer Institute* 90, no. 2 (1998).

Huang, Zhiping, et al.
Dual effects of weight and weight gain on breast cancer risk.
Journal of the American Medical Association 278, no. 17 (1997):
1407–1411.

Kumar, Nagi B.
Timing of weight gain and breast cancer risk.
Cancer 76, no. 2 (1995).

Weindruch, Richard, and Lisa Underhill.
Caloric intake and aging.
New England Journal of Medicine 337, no. 14.(1997): 986–994.

Daughters: Intergenerational Breast Cancer Prevention

Enger, S. M.
Breast-feeding history, pregnancy experience and risk of breast
cancer.
British Journal of Cancer 76, no. 1 (1997): 118–123.

Hankinson, Susan E.
Reproductive factors and family history of breast cancer in relation to plasma estrogen and prolactin levels in postmenopausal women in the Nurses Health Study.
Cancer Causes and Control 6 (1995): 217–224.

Kennedy, K .I.
Effects of breast-feeding on women's health.
International Journal of Gynecology and Obstetrics 47 (1994): S11–S20.

Kohlmeier, Lenore.
Future of dietary exposure assessment.
American Journal of Clinical Nutrition 61 (1995): 702S–709S.

Lourdes, Maria.
Effects of infant nutrition on cholesterol synthesis rates.
Pediatric Research 35, no. 2 (1994).

Murrill, W. B.
Prepubertal genistein exposure suppresses mammary cancer and enhances gland differentiation in rats.
Carcinogenesis 17, no. 77 (1996): 1451–1457.

SYMPOSIA

Reducing carcinogen levels in grilled chicken. American Chemical Society meetings, April 17, 1997.

Second international symposium on the role of soy in preventing and treating chronic disease. September 19, 1996. Brussels, Belgium.

BOOKS

Brumberg, Joan Jacobs. *The Body Project: An Intimate History of American Girls*. Random House, 1997.

Epstein, Samuel S,. and David Steinman with Suzanne Le Vert. *The Breast Cancer Prevention Program*. Macmillan, 1997.

Food, Nutrition and the Prevention of Cancer. World Cancer Research Fund and the American Institute for Cancer Research, 1997.

Jenkins, Nancy Harmon. *The Mediterranean Diet Cookbook*. Bantam, 1994.

Love, Susan M., M.D., with Karen Lindsey. *Dr. Susan Love's Hormone Book*. Random House, 1997.

Michnovicz, Jon J., and Diane S. Klein. *How to Reduce Your Risk of Breast Cancer*. Warner Books, 1996.

Simone, Charles B. *Breast Health*. Avery Publishing Group, 1995.

Simopoulos, Artemis P., and Jo Robinson. *The Omega Plan*. Harper-Collins, 1998.

US 1997 Soyfoods Directory.
Indiana Soybean Development Council.

NEWSLETTER

The Ribbon: A newsletter of the Cornell University Program on
Breast Cancer and Environmental Risk Factors in New York State

PROCEEDINGS

The Department of Defense. *Breast Cancer Research Program
Meeting Proceedings.* Volumes 1–2. October 31–November 4, 1997.

Index

251

Index

Index